AF812854

Rehabilitation in Diabetic Peripheral Neuropathy

Manu Goyal • Kanu Goyal
Editors

Rehabilitation in Diabetic Peripheral Neuropathy

Springer

Editors
Manu Goyal
Maharishi Markandeshwar Institute
of Physiotherapy and Rehabilitation
Maharishi Markandeshwar
(Deemed to be University)
Mullana - Ambala, Haryana, India

Kanu Goyal
Maharishi Markandeshwar Institute
of Physiotherapy and Rehabilitation
Maharishi Markandeshwar
(Deemed to be University)
Mullana - Ambala, Haryana, India

ISBN 978-981-97-9289-4 ISBN 978-981-97-9290-0 (eBook)
https://doi.org/10.1007/978-981-97-9290-0

© The Editor(s) (if applicable) and The Author(s), under exclusive license to Springer Nature Singapore Pte Ltd. 2024
This work is subject to copyright. All rights are solely and exclusively licensed by the Publisher, whether the whole or part of the material is concerned, specifically the rights of translation, reprinting, reuse of illustrations, recitation, broadcasting, reproduction on microfilms or in any other physical way, and transmission or information storage and retrieval, electronic adaptation, computer software, or by similar or dissimilar methodology now known or hereafter developed.
The use of general descriptive names, registered names, trademarks, service marks, etc. in this publication does not imply, even in the absence of a specific statement, that such names are exempt from the relevant protective laws and regulations and therefore free for general use.
The publisher, the authors and the editors are safe to assume that the advice and information in this book are believed to be true and accurate at the date of publication. Neither the publisher nor the authors or the editors give a warranty, expressed or implied, with respect to the material contained herein or for any errors or omissions that may have been made. The publisher remains neutral with regard to jurisdictional claims in published maps and institutional affiliations.

This Springer imprint is published by the registered company Springer Nature Singapore Pte Ltd.
The registered company address is: 152 Beach Road, #21-01/04 Gateway East, Singapore 189721, Singapore

If disposing of this product, please recycle the paper.

Foreword

युक्ताहारविहारस्य युक्तचेष्टस्य कर्मसु ।.
युक्तस्वप्नावबोधस्य योगो भवति दुःखहा ॥.
(Bhagavad Gita 6:17)

Diabetes mellitus is a growing worldwide health issue. This chronic and sometimes life-threatening condition affects millions of people. Annually, the disease claims the lives of around three million patients, and India is slowly becoming the world capital for diabetes. The enormous prevalence of diabetes worldwide necessitates proactive and adaptable approaches in terms of healthcare, health literacy, and public governance. The evolution of lifestyle from the past to the present where people are now indulged in sedentary behavior, unhealthy dietary patterns, poor-quality sleep, and stress has had a profound impact on health outcomes, particularly concerning the prevalence and management of chronic conditions like diabetes.

As mentioned in Bhagavad Gita shlok (mentioned above), "He who is temperate in his habits of eating, sleeping, working, and recreation can mitigate all material pains by practicing the yoga system." It emphasizes the importance of moderation and balance in various aspects of life, including diet (ahara), physical activity (vihar), work (karma), and rest (swapna). Following a balanced lifestyle, maintaining healthy habits, and practicing self-discipline can contribute to overall well-being, which is essential for effectively managing diabetes.

Diabetes is a metabolic disorder fueled in part by sedentary lifestyles and poor dietary choices. However, nestled within the folds of our cultural heritage are time-tested strategies for its prevention and control. Practices such as mindful eating, maintaining an optimal body weight, and observing an early dinner have long been revered in our traditional wisdom. Centuries before the advent of modern medicine, our ancestors intuitively recognized the profound connection between lifestyle and health. They followed the principles of "Satvik Ahar," emphasizing the consumption of wholesome, unprocessed foods abundant in nutrients. They embraced physical activity as an integral part of their daily routine, whether through agricultural labor, brisk walks, or yoga.

However, with the tide of westernization sweeping across societies, we have gradually drifted from these ancestral roots. Fast-paced lifestyles, characterized by processed foods, sedentary jobs, and erratic eating patterns, have become the new normal. As a result of our growing attraction to the Western way of life, we are losing the wonderful features of the Sanatan, Hindu, and Indian traditions. The repercussions are evident in the rising tide of chronic diseases, including diabetes, that afflict our communities. Yet, amid this tumult of change, there arises an opportunity for introspection. It is high time to rediscover the timeless wisdom encoded in our cultural heritage. It is high time to consider "जो पाया उसमें खो न जाएँ, जो खोया उसका ध्यान करें॥."

Diabetes if not managed in time can lead to complications, including ulcers, infections, and neuropathy, which are common yet preventable complications of diabetes; therefore, a dedicated book can educate individuals about the importance and strategies for the prevention and management of diabetes and its complications.

I would like to congratulate Prof (Dr.) Manu Goyal and Dr. Kanu Goyal, who possess great knowledge in the field of physiotherapy and who made the decision to publish a book on a topic that is frequently neglected.

I wholeheartedly recommend this book *Rehabilitation in Diabetic Peripheral Neuropathy* to readers seeking comprehensive knowledge and practical guidance in managing this critical aspect of diabetes. Whether you are a patient, caregiver, or healthcare professional, the insights and strategies outlined in this book will empower you to take proactive steps in preventing foot complications, promoting healing, and improving your overall well-being.

Department of Medicine, Maharishi Markandeshwar Institute of Medical Sciences and Research
Maharishi Markandeshwar (Deemed to be University),
Ambala, Haryana, India

Sunita Gupta

Preface

In the quest to understand and manage diabetic neuropathy, a condition that affects millions globally, we stand at the intersection of challenge and opportunity. This book, *Rehabilitation in Diabetic Peripheral Neuropathy*, is conceived from a deep desire to bridge the gap between medical understanding and practical management of one of diabetes' most complex and debilitating complications.

Diabetic neuropathy represents a spectrum of nerve disorders caused by diabetes. For those living with diabetes, neuropathy can be a source of significant discomfort, disability, and even life-threatening complications. The journey of managing diabetic neuropathy is often long, marked by trials and errors, and filled with a constant search for relief and functionality.

This book is written for patients, caregivers, and healthcare professionals. It aims to demystify the complexities of diabetic neuropathy, offering clear, concise, and practical guidance on its rehabilitation. We delve into the pathophysiology of diabetic neuropathy, elucidating how elevated blood sugar levels over time lead to nerve damage. Understanding the "why" behind the condition is the first step in confronting it.

Following this, we explore the "how" of managing diabetic neuropathy through rehabilitation strategies. The focus is on practical approaches to pain management, physical therapy, and lifestyle modifications. Each chapter is crafted to provide actionable advice, grounded in the latest research and clinical practices, yet presented in a way that is accessible to all readers.

A unique feature of this book is its emphasis on the holistic management of diabetic neuropathy. Beyond the physical symptoms, diabetic neuropathy can take a toll on emotional well-being. Thus, we include chapters dedicated to coping strategies, mental health considerations, and the importance of a supportive community in the rehabilitation process.

Our contributors are esteemed professionals from across the spectrum of diabetes care and rehabilitation. Their insights offer a well-rounded perspective on the challenges and advancements in treating diabetic neuropathy. Through their expertise, we bring forward a guide that is both informative and empathetic, recognizing the individual experiences of those living with diabetic neuropathy.

As you turn these pages, our hope is that you will find not only information but also inspiration. The path to managing diabetic neuropathy is not one walked alone. This book is a companion for that journey, offering guidance, support, and the reassurance that, though the road may be difficult, there are steps we can take toward improvement and better quality of life.

Rehabilitation in Diabetic Peripheral Neuropathy is more than a guide; it is a testament to the resilience of the human spirit in the face of chronic illness. It is a call to action for more compassionate, comprehensive care for those affected. Welcome to a resource that we hope will enlighten, encourage, and empower you or your loved ones to navigate the complexities of diabetic neuropathy with confidence and hope.

Ambala, Haryana, India Manu Goyal
Ambala, Haryana, India Kanu Goyal

Contents

Chapter 1
Diabetic Peripheral Neuropathy

Parul Sharma

Contents

1.1 Introduction

Worldwide, diabetes is a severe chronic illness that significantly lowers people's quality of life. With an expected 4 million deaths globally in 2017, it is among the top 10 leading causes of mortality for adults [1]. According to the International Diabetes Federation (IDF), the global prevalence of diabetes mellitus (DM) in 20–79-year-olds in 2021 was estimated to be 536.6 million people, rising to 783.2

P. Sharma (✉)
School of Physiotherapy, Delhi Pharmaceutical Sciences & Research University, New Delhi, India
e-mail: parul_sharma.dpsru@dpsru.edu.in

© The Author(s), under exclusive license to Springer Nature Singapore Pte Ltd. 2024

M. Goyal, K. Goyal (eds.), *Rehabilitation in Diabetic Peripheral Neuropathy*,
https://doi.org/10.1007/978-981-97-9290-0_1

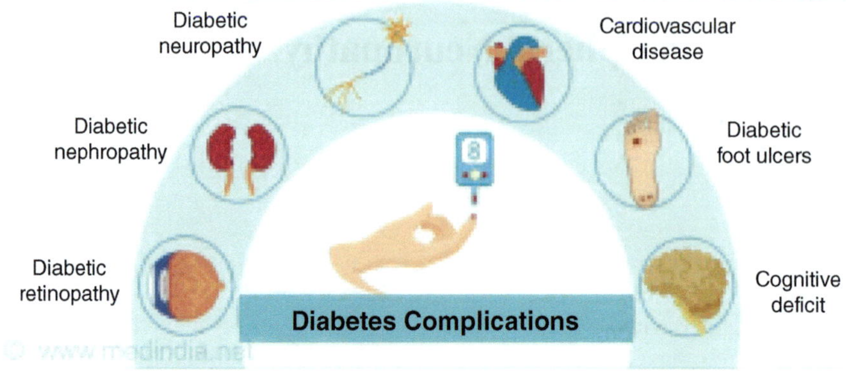

Fig. 1.1 Complications of diabetes mellitus. (From https://images.app.goo.gl/CEv3S1FTd-vnwmoYn9)

million in 2045 [2]. Globally, around 3 million deaths annually are due to DM, and 49.7% live with diabetes undiagnosed [3].

There are 88 million diabetics in the South-East Asian region, 77 million of whom live in India. Type 2 diabetes mellitus (T2DM) has become a major threat to public health and affects individuals of all ages [4]. Diabetic neuropathy is the most common chronic microvascular complication of diabetes, with diabetic peripheral neuropathy (DPN) affecting nearly 50% of diabetes patients over their lifetime [5–7]. DPN leads to neuropathic pain, foot ulceration, infections, and amputation, which place a large burden on diabetes care worldwide [8]. Clinicians need to watch out for complications in these patients because type 2 diabetes is a chronic condition and young patients are more likely to develop diabetic neuropathy. Because of its complications, diabetes results in higher rates of death, illness, incapacity, and monetary loss when compared to other chronic illnesses (Fig. 1.1). The American Diabetes Association defines peripheral nerve dysfunction (DPN) as the presence of symptoms and/or indicators in individuals with DM [9].

DPN is one of the most common and dangerous microvascular complications associated with diabetes. Peripheral nerve injury is primarily caused by DPN, making diabetics more likely to experience impairment and lowering their quality of life. Uncertainty persists, nevertheless, regarding the global frequency and risk factors of DPN, particularly in low- and middle-income nations [10].

1.2 Epidemiology

The prevalence of diabetes is predicted to rise from 9.3% (463 million) in 2019 to 10.2% (578 million) by 2030 and 10.9% (700 million) by 2045 worldwide. Globally, diabetes is now considered to be an epidemic. The International Diabetes Federation estimates that 425 million people worldwide had diabetes in 2017, and by 2045, that figure is predicted to increase to 628 million (Fig. 1.2). The frequency of diabetic complications will also climb in tandem with this increase. It is believed that almost half of those with diabetes have DPN, which is the most frequent cause of neuropathy globally. It raises mortality, lowers quality of life, and produces significant morbidity [11]. There has been a rise in both the prevalence of diabetes and the incidence of chronic diabetic complications. Diabetes frequently results in diabetic peripheral neuropathies (DPNs), which are chronic conditions. Distal symmetric polyneuropathy (DSPN), the most common type of DPN, affects at least 20% of people with type 1 diabetes and almost 50% of patients with type 2 diabetes after 10 years. Moreover, 20–25% of people with type 2 diabetes who receive a new diagnosis may also be diagnosed with DSPN. About 15–30% of all diabetes patients have unpleasant DPN, even though the great majority of DPN patients do not experience any discomfort [12, 13]. Type 1 and type 2 diabetes have different prevalence rates of diabetes-related pancreatic cancer (DPN), with low rates in newly diagnosed individuals rising to 34% after 25 years (Diabetic Control and Complications Trial, DCCT). The EURODIAB IDDM is the European Insulin-Dependent Diabetes Mellitus Prospective Complications study, which involved 16 European nations, and found comparable rates. The results of contemporary cohort data from the American and Atlantic cohorts are likewise comparable. Throughout their lives, Over 50% of individuals with type 2 diabetes report having DPN symptoms; even in newly diagnosed and early cases, rates can reach 20–30%. This prevalence is high, as documented in large observational or interventional cohorts, including the ADDITION trial and GRADE (Glycemia Reduction Approaches in Diabetes–A Comparative Effectiveness) trials, where over 1500 individuals with screen-detected type 2 diabetes were studied [14]. Most research studies don't differentiate between patients

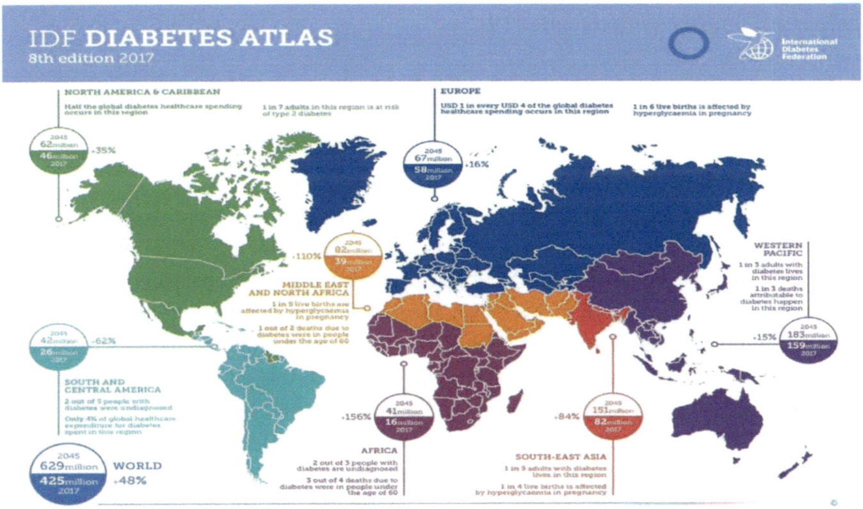

Fig. 1.2 Epidemiology of diabetes mellitus. (From https://images.app.goo.gl/UyYMKWD1Y-iwyMJKK6)

with diabetes of types I and II. Another Knowledge gap is the current study's area of interest regarding the risk factors that result in diabetic neuropathy. DPN screenings for pre-diabetes are uncommon, despite indications of a high DPN prevalence rate beginning at the time of T2D diagnosis. Due to delayed diagnosis in the majority of T2D patients, the precise period of diabetes development is difficult to pinpoint. So, it's still unclear what changes connected to polyneuropathy over time [15].

Cornerstones of intervention efforts to avoid DPN-related consequences include early diagnosis and identification of at-risk persons. The magnitude of the issue, both personally and societally, necessitates a deeper comprehension of the illness to develop mechanism-based targets as well as an early diagnosis to avoid negative patient outcomes. Unfortunately, we still don't fully comprehend the etiology of DPN. As a result, there are no pharmacotherapies that can effectively change the illness and treat the condition. The cornerstone of modern care is reducing risk factors for DPN and preventing and controlling its effects [16]. The American Diabetes Association (ADA) claims that every patient should have a DPN evaluation beginning with the diagnosis of T2D and continuing annually for an additional 5 years following the diagnosis of T1D. Unfortunately, other than a healthier lifestyle and better diabetes management, there are no modifiable therapies for DN despite decades of study [17]. Despite this challenge, research on diabetic neuropathy has focused for the past 20 years on the T1D rat as the initial study model to be used for glucose investigate the development of diabetes. No treatment trials in the United States have been able to stop DN from progressing in its current form. Due to our inadequate knowledge of the condition, major pharmaceutical companies are now abandoning DPN, regardless of the problem is approaching epidemic proportions [18]. Similar to this, although there are certain distinctions between painful and painless DPN, the precise processes producing the disorder are yet unclear. Painful DPN is not commonly treated with disease-modifying medications, and the focus of care is still mostly symptomatic [19].

1.3 Etiology

In the United States and Europe, type 2 diabetes (T2D) and pre-diabetes are the most common causes of peripheral neuropathy. Every diabetic, including those with Type 1 diabetes (T1D), eventually develops neuropathy. The prevalence of type 2 diabetes (T2D) and pre-diabetes is on the rise, especially in countries that have adopted a more Westernized diet [20]. Persistently high blood serum glucose levels seem to cause tiny blood vessels to become damaged, this jeopardizes the neurons' ability to get oxygen and nourishment. The distal sensory and autonomic nerve fibers are first compromised, and as the damage moves closer to the site, the adaptive response of the foot joints and epidermis gradually declines. Asymmetric diabetic peripheral neuropathies may make up half of the cases. If patients' unresponsive feet go unnoticed and protective foot care is not given, they are more likely to sustain injuries [21]. Although there are many possible causes of DPN is the most prevalent kind of peripheral neuropathy, and can have detrimental effects. Early detection of peripheral polyneuropathy symptoms can help prevent neuropathic foot ulcers, which can cause mortality, septicemia, local to systemic infection, and limb damage. This reduces the risk of death and disability driven by the pathophysiologic failure of wound healing. What specifically caused DPN is not certain. Theories have been put up for the metabolic, neurovascular, and immunological pathways. Genetics, social, and lifestyle variables including smoking and heavy alcohol use have also been linked to mechanical compression (such as carpal tunnel syndrome) and genetic compression [22]. The most prevalent clinical category of etiologies that contribute to extremities pain from PN diseases is metabolic abnormalities. Although there are several potential causes of PN, DM is the most typical one. The following are some potential root reasons to consider:

- Nutritional deficits (such as a lack of B12 and a surplus of B6).
- Guillain-Barre syndrome, toxins (chemotherapy), and overdosing, hereditary or genetic disorders (such as porphyria, amyloidosis, and Charcot Marie Tooth disease), Infections (HIV), inflammatory diseases (like rheumatoid arthritis and lupus), hypothyroidism, and cancer.
- Age, high blood pressure, peripheral arterial disease, hyperlipidemia, poor glucose control, and heavy alcohol use are risk factors for PN (Fig. 1.3) [23].

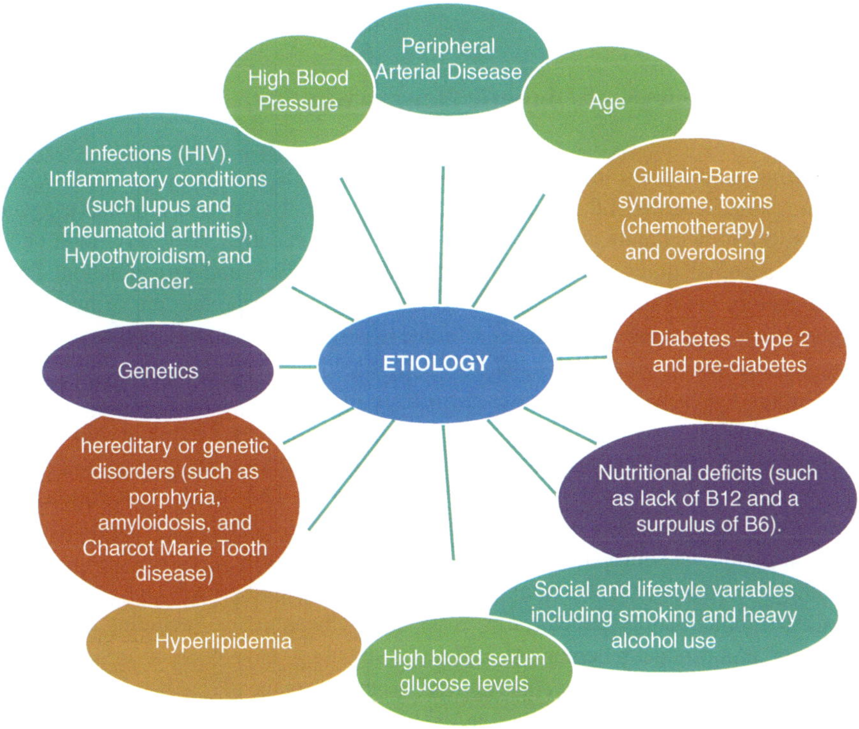

Fig. 1.3 Etiology of diabetic peripheral neuropathy. (From Schreiber et al. [23])

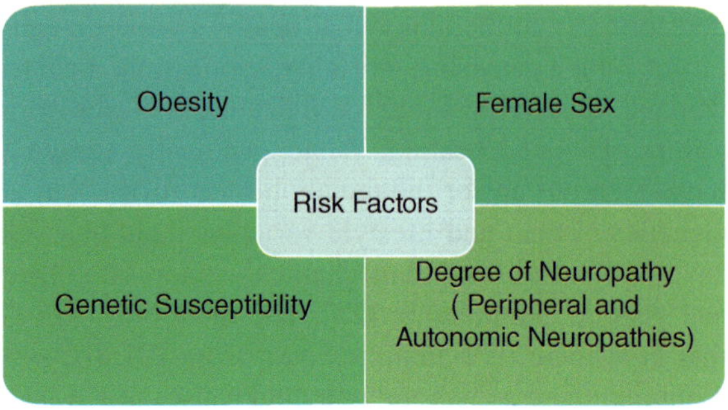

Fig. 1.4 Risk factors of diabetic peripheral neuropathy. (From Rossboth et al. [24])

1.4 Risk Factors

Numerous risk variables, including the degree of neuropathy, the burden of hyperglycemia, and obesity, have been proposed as causes of painful DPN. However, new research has shown compelling evidence linking the female sex to painful DPN. Risk factors for diabetes include obesity and genetic susceptibility. One of the main factors contributing to serious consequences of DM is peripheral and autonomic neuropathies (Fig. 1.4). A diabetic patient who develops a diabetic foot ulcer over 5 years has a 2.5-fold increased risk of passing away compared to a diabetic patient who does not [24].

1.5 Pathogenesis of Diabetic Neuropathy

Peripheral nerve damage in DPN is caused by a variety of mechanisms; the most important are oxidative stress, inflammation, and mitochondrial dysfunction. Diabetes triggers the activation of inflammatory molecules that lead to oxidative stress, glycation end-product accumulation, a functional nitric monoxide deficit, and inflammation. Pro-inflammatory cytokines such as TNF-, IL-6, and C-reactive protein are expressed at higher levels in patients with diabetes. Chronic hyperglycemia causes cytokines to infiltrate vascular tissue, which will reduce the body's ability to heal on its own [25].

Chronic hyperglycemia increases the release of cytokines by stimulating macrophages, which secrete TNF-. Atherosclerosis is accelerated by TNF-induced upregulation of endothelial cell adhesion molecules. In patients with poorly controlled diabetes, insulin resistance is worsened by increased TNF production caused by hyperglycemia. The effect of TNF- on Schwann cells also explains local demyelination in peripheral neuropathy [26]. Hyperglycemia primarily affects Schwann cells, resulting in cell damage, altered axon integrity, and impaired growth factor signaling. Defective inflammatory pathways in axons and Schwann cells, including advanced glycation end-product/receptor (AGE/RAGE) signaling, have been observed in diabetic neuropathy in animal models that lead to nerve damage [27]. An explanation for the loss of feeling in the distribution noted in DPN in the glove and stocking regions can be found in a study that used both animal and human models. Early damage to the distal axons of both upper and lower limb neurons has been associated with sensory neurodegeneration in the chronic stage of diabetes. These changes are accompanied by widespread defects in electrophysiology and gene expression, all of which contribute to a degenerative phenotype [28]. The information that is currently available on the development of DPN takes into consideration a variety of mRNA modifications that change the patterns of miRNA expression, leading to a range of DPN phenotypes. Among these changes are polyol accumulation, aberrant AGE-RAGE signaling, increased oxidative and nitric oxide stress, microangiopathy, and/or mitochondrial dysfunction. Dysfunction of endothelial nitric oxide synthase (eNOS) may be a major factor in the pathogenic cascade leading to complications of diabetic peripheral vascular disease (DPN). Therefore, it is thought that eNOS may have a role in the development of DPN. In the early stages of DPN, hyperglycemia is linked to abnormalities in the vasa nervorum and nerve fiber loss. The ischemia and hypoxia in the nerves of patients with T2DM due to microangiopathy of vasa nervorum have always been observed and possibly a pathogenic mechanism of DPN [29].

1.6 Classification of Diabetic Neuropathies

Fig. 1.5 and Table 1.1 describe the classification first proposed by PK Thomas [30] and modified in a recent Position Statement by the American Diabetes Association [31].

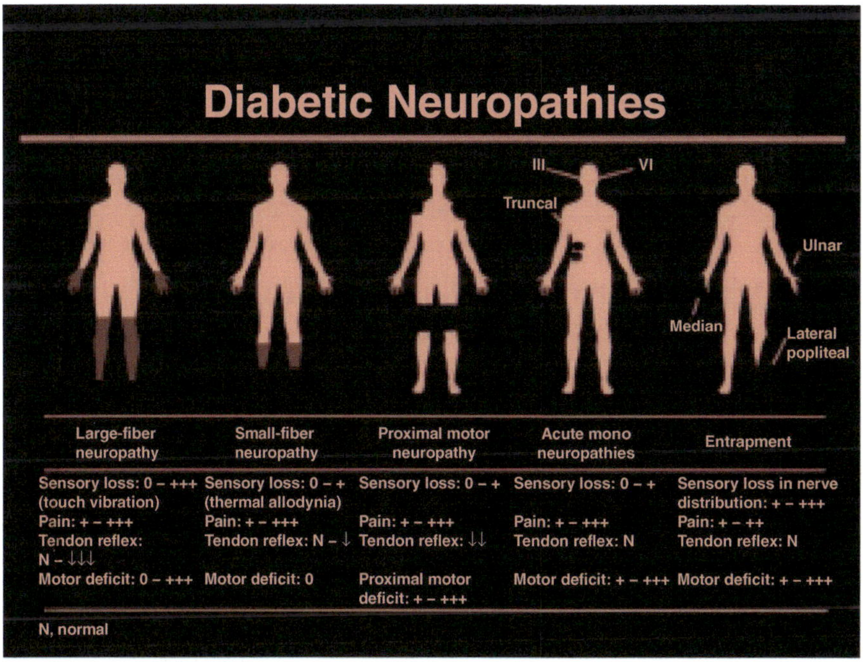

Fig. 1.5 Classification of diabetic neuropathies proposed by PK Thomas. (From Thomas [30])

Table 1.1 Classification of diabetic neuropathies proposed by PK Thomas

A.
Diffuse neuropathy
Distal symmetrical peripheral neuropathy
Primarily small-fiber neuropathy
Primarily large-fiber neuropathy
Mixed small- and large-fiber neuropathy (most common)
Autonomic
Cardiovascular
Reduced heart rate variability
Resting tachycardia
Orthostatic hypotension
Sudden death (malignant arrhythmia)
Gastrointestinal
Diabetic gastroparesis (gastropathy)
Diabetic enteropathy (diarrhea)
Colonic hypomotility (constipation)
Urogenital
Diabetic cytopathic (neurogenic bladder)
Erectile dysfunction
Female sexual dysfunction
Sudomotor dysfunction
Distal hypohidrosis/anhidrosis,
Gustatory sweating
Hypoglycemia
Abnormal pupillary function
B. Mononeuropathy (mononeuritis multiplex) (atypical forms)
Isolated cranial or peripheral nerve (e.g., Cranial Nerve III, ulnar, median, femoral, peroneal)
Mononeuritis multiplex (if confluent may resemble polyneuropathy)
C. Radiculopathy or polyradiculopathy (atypical forms)
Radiculoplexus neuropathy (a.k.a. lumbosacral polyradiculopathy, proximal motor amyotrophy)
Thoracic radiculopathy
D. Nondiabetic neuropathies common in diabetes
Pressure palsies
Chronic inflammatory demyelinating polyneuropathy
Radiculoplexus neuropathy
Acute painful small-fiber neuropathies (treatment-induced)

From Thomas [30]

1.7 Clinical Features of Diabetic Neuropathy

Numerous clinical indications and symptoms may accompany DPN. Some people may have no symptoms at all, in which case a foot ulcer may be the only sign. However, some individuals may encounter one or more symptoms, such as paresthesia, numbness, and neuropathic pain, which can range in severity from barely bothersome to unmanageable and result in severe suffering [32]. These symptoms might be intermittent or persistent, and each patient's natural course is unique. In addition to the usual involvement of the feet, it can cause a broader range of symptoms and signs, such as myelopathy-like, myopathy-like, and even fatal symptoms. Between 23% and 76% of people have diabetic neuropathy. Poor glycemic control, aging, chronic diabetes, visceral obesity, hypertension, smoking, dyslipidemia, and hyperinsulinemia are all associated with the advancement of DPN. In the first year of their diabetes, 5–10% of patients develop neuropathy; 20 years later, 60–70% of diabetic patients have some kind of DPN [33]. Sensory sensations could only last a short while before going away totally, or they might persist for a long time. Sensory complaints and clinical examination indicators start symmetrically in the toes and distal foot. Physical examination findings often show that the distal foot is initially affected by light touch and pinpricking. This is often followed by more severe motor and sensory impairments (e.g., loss of proprioception and vibration) as well as symptoms of weakness, toe clawing, loss of ankle reflex, and loss of muscle mass. The sickness initially affects the tips of the fingers and upper limbs before moving proximally up the leg as the condition worsens. Patients with painful DPN are typically not distinguished from those without neuropathic pain during the physical examination. The loss of small-fiber modalities (such as temperature and pinprick sensations) may occur in certain people with pure small-fiber neuropathy, despite normal big fiber function. Clinically, asymmetric sensory alterations may be present in approximately half of patients with DPN. A small subset of patients also exhibits the so-called "irritable nociceptor" phenotype, which is characterized by "positive" sensory symptoms such as allodynia and hyperalgesia. Peripheral nerve system (PNS) damage can result from diabetes in several ways (Tables 1.2a and 1.2b). The stocking-glove variety of nerve damage is the most prevalent. Damage to the foot nerves that is symmetrical, bilateral, and worsens from the proximal to the distal regions is the condition's hallmark. Due to the frequency with which this pattern of nerve damage occurs, this neuropathy is referred to as diabetic neuropathy (DN). It is thought that the damage to nerves induced by diabetes has become an ongoing process ranging from normal glycemia to varying degrees of hyperglycemia is supported by the pattern of injury observed in prediabetes [33, 34].

Table 1.2a Clinical manifestations of small and large fiber neuropathies

Clinical signs of neuropathies in the small fibers:
Aδ and C fibers that are not myelinated and have thin myelination are impacted.
Severe symptoms, including hyperalgesia, dysesthesia, and allodynia, frequently accompanied by burning, superficial, or lancinating pain.
The development of numbness and hypoalgesia (progression of neuropathy must be carefully ruled out by examination; the absence of pain may not always indicate nerve death rather than nerve recovery).
Abnormal thermal perception of warmth and cold.
Abnormal autonomic function characterized by cold feet, dry skin, reduced sweating, and impaired vasomotion and skin blood flow.
Reflexes in the deep tendons and intact motor strength.
Findings of negative nerve conduction velocity.
Cutaneous nerve fiber loss observed during skin biopsies.
Using the Wartenberg wheel or a comparable device, prickling pain perception and decreased responsiveness to 1.0 g one can use Semmes Weinstein monofilament to reach a clinical diagnosis.
People who could develop foot ulcers, which could lead to cause gangrene and require amputations.

From Anandhanarayanan et al. [34]

Table 1.2b Clinical manifestations of small and large fiber neuropathies

Clinical signs of neuropathies in the large fibers:
Both motor and sensory nerves may be affected by the large myelinated rapidly conducting Aα/β fibers that are affected.
Prominent symptoms include sensory ataxia (duckling gait), small intrinsic muscle wasting in the hands and feet, hammertoe deformities, and hand and foot weakness.
Abnormal reflexes in deep tendon.
Impaired joint position perception, light touch, and vibration perception—often the first objective indication.
Pes equinus causes the Achilles tendon to shorten.
Minimal symptoms could include feeling as though you're walking on cotton, "strange" floors, not being able to turn pages in a book, or not being able to tell one coin from another. Some patients are unable to stand on their toes or heels due to severe distal muscle weakness.
Findings of abnormal nerve conduction velocity
Patients with hot feet have increased skin blood flow.
Patients who are more likely to fall, break, or develop Charcot Neuroarthropathy
Nonetheless, most DPN patients have a "mixed" form of neuropathy, which results in damage to both large and small nerve fibers.

From Anandhanarayanan et al. [34]

1.8 DPN and Pain Diagnosis

DPN can be diagnosed at the bedside with careful clinical examination of the feet and legs using simple tools within a few minutes. An examination of the feet, a neurological examination of sensation using basic semi-quantitative bedside instruments like the 10 g Semmes-Weinstein monofilament, Neuropen (to assess

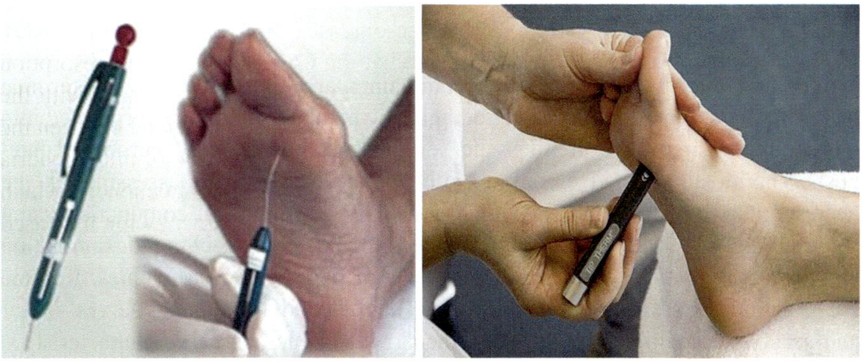

Fig. 1.6a Neuropen with 1 10 g monofilament & 1 Neurotip NeuroQuick or Tiptherm (temperature). (From https://images.app.goo.gl/YLWJB3YViewZcbMq5)

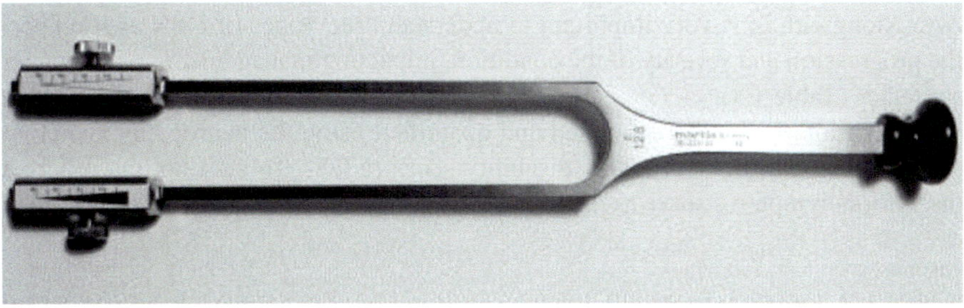

Fig. 1.6b Rydel-Seiffer tuning fork (vibration). (From https://images.app.goo.gl/51S9xA4dyUMe8fPF9)

Table 1.3 Examination—Bedside sensory tests

Sensory modality	Nerve fiber	Instrument	Associated sensory receptors
Vibration	Aβ (large)	128 HzTuning fork	Ruffini corpuscle mechanoreceptors
Pain (pinprick)	C (small)	Neuro-tips	Nociceptors for pain and warmth
Pressure	Aβ, Aα (large)	1 g and 10 gMonofilament	Pacinian corpuscle
Light touch	Aβ, Aα (large)	Wisp of cotton	Meissner's corpuscle
Cold	Aδ (small)	Cold tuning fork	Cold thermoreceptors

From Bajwa and Khalili [36]

touch/pressure), NeuroQuick or Tiptherm (temperature) (Fig. 1.6a), calibrated Rydel-Seiffer tuning fork (vibration) (Fig. 1.6b), pinprick (pain), and tendon reflexes (knee and ankle) are all part of the basic neurological assessment (Table 1.3). In addition, the assessment of joint position and motor power should also be assessed [35].

1.9 Assessment of DPN

Nerve conduction studies, subjective complaints, and signs are used to determine the prevalence of neuropathy. Electrodiagnostic results should be incorporated into the evaluation since they offer a greater level of specificity in polyneuropathy diagnosis. The most informative component of the electrodiagnostic assessment is the nerve conduction study (NCS), which is usually performed in conjunction using electromyography with a needle. NCSs have long been the benchmark examination or standard by which to verify the diagnosis of peripheral neuropathies. Routine NCSs include assessment of the tibial, sural, median, radial, and ulnar nerves' motor and sensory capacities in addition to their own. Numerous nerve characteristics, including amplitudes, latencies, conduction velocities, and F-wave latencies as functions of myelination, are used to assess axonal status. Axonal damage causes amplitudes to decrease. Demyelinating neuropathies are characterized by prolonged longer F-wave latencies, slower conduction velocities, and nerve conduction latencies. Alongwith, it is very important to understand the stages of DPN as it reflects the progression and severity of the condition, impacting management and treatment strategies (Table 1.4).

In addition, DPN was examined and quantified using the neuropathy symptom score (NSS) and the neuropathy disability score (NDS). To sum up, the reported discomfort symptoms serve as the foundation for the NSS. Considerations included

Table 1.4 A staging system, which has four stages, was used to provide a framework for the diagnosis and management of DPN

Stage of diabetic peripheral neuropathy	Characteristics
Stages 0/1	No clinical neuropathy Asymptomatic
Stage 2	
a) Chronic Painful	Positive symptomatology nocturnal pain, burning, shooting, stabbing pains ± pins, and needles It may have absent sensation to several modalities and reduced or absent reflexes Less common
b) Acute Painful	It may be associated with the initiation of glycemic therapy in poorly controlled diabetes Normal or minor sensory features in the peripheral neurological examination
c) Painless with complete/partial sensory loss	No symptoms or numbness/deadness of feet; reduced thermal sensitivity; painless injury Signs of reduced or absent sensation with absence of reflexes
Stage 3 Late complications of clinical neuropathy	Foot lesions, e.g., ulcers Neuropathic deformity, e.g., Charcot joint nontraumatic amputation

From Yang et al. [35]

the location, timing, and potential relief (e.g., nocturnal awakening) of the symptoms, as well as the burning, numbness, tingling (2p), fatigue, and cramping and aching feelings (1p). The NSS was divided into three groups: moderate (score: 5–6), severe (score: 7–10), and mild (score: 3–4).NDS was created by a neurological examination that measured vibration, temperature, pain, and the reflex of the Achilles tendon in both feet. To determine the overall disability score, each test was assigned a point value (up to a maximum of 10). DPN diagnosis was based on the co-occurrence of signs and symptoms. According to the national guidelines, we defined DPN as at least moderate signs (NDS $\geq$6) with or without symptoms or mild signs (NDS $\geq$3) with moderate symptoms (NSS $\geq$5) [36–38].

1.10 Physiotherapy Treatment

Adverse outcomes can be avoided with improved glycemic control, early detection, and preventive care. Nutritionists, endocrinologists, neurologists, pain specialists, nurse practitioners, podiatrists, psychologists, physiotherapists, and other specialists should ideally be included in a multidisciplinary team. Most people concur that the first line of treatment for any kind of diabetic neuropathy should be strict blood glucose control. Not only are hypertension and hyperlipidemia prevalent in DPN, but they also pose a risk for large vessel diseases and need to be managed. As first-line treatments, the European Federation of Neurological Societies advises using TCAs, SNRIs, gabapentin, or pregabalin. There are wide ranges of alternative therapies available for DPN pain, which include acupuncture, near-infrared phototherapy, low-intensity laser therapy, transcutaneous electrical stimulation, frequency-modulated electromagnetic neural stimulation therapy, high-frequency external muscle stimulation, and as a last resort, the implantation of an electrical spinal cord stimulator [38, 39].

As neuropathy progresses, the foot's dynamic stability, mobility, and capacity for locomotor tasks are all compromised by the weakening of the neural structures, muscles, and joints—particularly the tiny joints and intrinsic muscles of the foot and ankle. When a patient is walking, all of these losses affect how the load is absorbed and transmitted, putting the foot at risk for mechanical overloads that damage the tissue and lower the quality of life. Treatment for diabetes patients is usually passive. Relieving plantar load is only recommended when the consequences of severe neuropathy, such as ulcerations, amputations, and deformed feet, are already apparent. Active and preventive therapeutic actions, on the other hand, are strongly recommended for delaying or even preventing sensory, motor, and tissue complications, thus reducing the effect of disease on quality of life [40].

Three important interventions are thought to be necessary for diabetic patients: diet, exercise, and medication [41]. Diabetes is widely recognized in patients' lipid metabolism, cardiovascular risk factors, and glucose control all improve with exercise therapy. However, researchers cannot agree on what comprises an ideal exercise program [42].

Conversely, compared to healthy individuals, those who have diabetes have lower activity rates. Consequently, it is necessary to provide safe and vigorous training as well as motivation techniques to encourage participation in longer-term programs for training. Numerous research has looked at the benefits of Tai Chi, aerobic, functional, weight-bearing, non-weight-bearing, strengthening, and stretching activities for diabetic patients [43]. Multimodal mind-body exercise like tai chi incorporates social, psychological, cognitive, and physical elements. It is becoming more and more popular. Exercises including tai chi have been demonstrated to have a good impact on lipid metabolism, glucose regulation, and lower extremity microcirculation. Improvements in glucose metabolism after Tai Chi activities can be linked to recovery, which lowers HbA1c levels and insulin resistance [42, 43].

However, a systematic review research discovered conflicting findings about how Tai Chi workouts affect glucose regulation. This might be because various studies used varied Tai Chi exercise types, durations, and intensities. Tai Chi activities have been shown by Wang et al. [44] to have a favorable impact on peripheral sensory function. After doing Tai Chi exercises, they found that diabetes patients' skin had more blood volume. Research from the past has indicated that practicing Tai Chi has positive effects. Individuals with somatic limitations and diabetes can confidently follow and execute these processes [45].

Protocols for progressive resistance training are particularly useful for building muscle. They can also aid in reducing pain and disability and building muscle mass. Patients with DPN have been found to benefit from exercises for their ankles and feet in terms of lower extremity function, plantar pressure during gait, and daily activities. The structure and function of the foot benefit from exercises that strengthen the entire body while exercises that improve ankle and foot flexibility and strength can help reduce pain and disability. However, the ankle and the intrinsic muscles of the foot are disregarded in these exercises. Exercise logbooks and pedometers are examples of scheduled walking instruction that is coupled with an observation component in a home-based exercise treatment program. It may be claimed that stretching activities, both active and passive, increased ankle joint mobility while lowering peak pressure in diabetes individuals. For a month, these exercises were done three times a day, with a ten-second rest period between each joint position. Patients with DPN might benefit from practical and helpful general activities that enhance balance. Time-space gait characteristics increase with a particular training program that incorporates circuit and balancing exercises, as demonstrated by Allet et al. [46] in their RCT study. Improvement in these individuals' neuromuscular control and plantar sensation can be linked to improvements after balancing training. Home exercise improves the mobility of the foot joints and balances plantar pressure during stride, according to studies [45, 47].

Weight-bearing exercise consists of two weekly units: 15 min of intense exercise and 30 min of moderate exercise. For people with DPN, weight-bearing exercises—which typically involve walking and don't call for specialized gear—are crucial because they maintain their overall fitness, bone health, and mobility. One study found that individuals with DPN who took part in a low-intensity walking program increased their daily walking mileage without seeing an increase in wounds.

Individuals who do not have severe foot abnormalities or open ulcers should adhere to a program that can be made to be either weight-bearing or non-weight-bearing to satisfy their individual needs. Large muscle groups and repeated motions are characteristics of aerobic activities, which also raise heart rate slightly and lower the risk of chronic disease. During aerobic exercise, increased shear stress is favorable and may help the artery wall's adaptive structural changes [48]. Research indicates that by enhancing overall vascular health, moderate-intensity aerobic exercise lowers the risk of cardiovascular disease. DPN interferes with nerve degeneration, which can have an impact on flow-mediated dilation and other vascular measures. According to one study, 16 weeks of aerobic exercise increased maximum arterial diameter and accelerated the speed of the reaction to maximal dilatation [42].

1.10.1 Electrotherapy

Electrotherapy interventions include low-level laser therapy, plantar electrical stimulation, and percutaneous electrical nerve stimulation (PENS). This section discusses each of these treatments and their outcomes. Plantar electrical stimulation is the process of stimulating the plantar surface with an electrotherapy device. An RCT research has demonstrated that using plantar electrical stimulation regularly is a non-invasive, secure, and successful method of helping people with DPN improve their motor function [42].

Improved plantar skin perfusion is thought to be the cause of individuals with DPN experiencing an improvement in plantar sensation after daily electrical stimulation. As previously mentioned by Malik et al. [49], decreased local blood flow in DPN patients may result in oxidative stress and the production of substances that impede the transmission of nerve impulses. In a systematic review study involving 21 RCT publications, researchers used electrical stimulation to treat wounds and demonstrated its many benefits, including enhanced skin perfusion through the production of vascular endothelial growth factor. The healing of the foot ulcers and subsequent improved blood flow resulting from plantar electrical stimulation may be the cause of recovery. In one study, individuals with DPN who used electric stimulation daily for 6 weeks saw a greater improvement in their balance than those who did balancing exercises [50].

Electroacupuncture is a technique used to treat energy imbalances in the body by introducing needles into various body parts. A novel electroanalgesic treatment called transcutaneous electrical nerve stimulation, also known as PENS, combines electroacupuncture with TENS to treat peripheral neuropathy and pain. Peripheral sensory nerves in the region of neuropathic pain are stimulated by PENS, and the cumulative benefits over time suggest long-term effects. While the exact process that causes analgesia is still, it may have to do with elevated concentrations of substances similar to opioids in the central nervous system as well as neural modulation. Studies by Cameron et al. [51] and Mo et al. [52] showed that electrical stimulation played a significant role in normalizing neural conduction velocity in animal samples. Diabetes-related foot ulcers can also be treated with low-level laser treatment. This particular laser type has potential benefits, including decreased pain signals, improved blood flow, and anti-inflammatory effects. Numerous studies have demonstrated the efficacy of low-level laser therapy in managing nerve regeneration. It has also been shown to have an impact on diabetic mellitus patients who suffer from excruciating DPN.

Low-level laser therapy was used in one study to relieve the pain of DPN patients. The release of cytokines and circulating growth factors, which promote vasodilation and the development of new capillaries, maybe one reason for this. Alternatively, it could have been caused by increased microcirculation. Patients with diabetic neuropathy may benefit from laser therapy among electrotherapy techniques because it damages the nervous system and treats neurological diseases [53].

1.10.2 Foot Care

Reducing tissue stress is thought to be the primary objective of interventions for neuropathy patients. These are accomplished by prescribing footwear, orthotics with rocker soles, and specially-made insoles. These orthotic devices' main goal is to alter the rolling gait of the foot to passively reallocate plantar pressure. However, due to enhanced joint stability and muscle function, active foot loading adjustment during foot and ankle exercise therapy may improve force absorption and transmission. Therefore, it is advised to use an orthotic device to prevent foot ulcers in addition to a therapeutic exercise program to enhance the functional ability of the affected foot [54].

1.11 Conclusion

Individuals with DM who are not treated or whose medication is not appropriate may experience more serious consequences. Frequently, neuropathy is the cause of skin degeneration, ulcer formation, and infection. Amputations of the limbs and toes are not uncommon. Unfortunately, the majority of instances of diabetic neuropathy therapy fail, and there are still problems with it. A complete cure for neuropathy symptoms is common. Autonomic neuropathy patients with DM frequently have greater fatality rates, especially if they also have heart problems. Although the overall fatality rates over 10 years vary from 15% to 30%, amputation of a limb also results in significant sickness. Diabetic neuropathy, which can present as either painful or non-painful, can be brought on by type 2 diabetes. The non-painful variety is the most deadly due to its stealthy nature and progressive loss of feeling in the feet and lower limbs. As a result, patients with neuropathy are more likely to experience limb amputation, foot ulcers, and deformities because they may not receive a diagnosis until irreversible nerve damage has occurred. Therefore, it is essential to recognize DN early. The best approach to managing diabetes, in general, is to recommend routinely doing basic screening tests to potentially prevent more neuronal damage.

References

1. Saeedi P, Petersohn I, Salpea P, Malanda B, Karuranga S, Unwin N, et al. Global and regional diabetes prevalence estimates for 2019 and projections for 2030 and 2045: results from the International Diabetes Federation Diabetes Atlas, 9th edition. Diabetes Res Clin Pract. 2019;157:107843. https://doi.org/10.1016/j.diabres.2019.107843.
2. Sun H, Saeedi P, Karuranga S, Pinkepank M, Ogurtsova K, Duncan BB, et al. IDF Diabetes Atlas: global, regional, and country-level diabetes prevalence estimates for 2021 and projections for 2045. Diabetes Res Clin Pract. 2022;183:109119. https://doi.org/10.1016/j.diabres.2021.109119.
3. Cho NH, Shaw JE, Karuranga S, Huang Y, et al. IDF Diabetes Atlas: global estimates of diabetes prevalence for 2017 and projections for 2045. Diabetes Res Clin Pract. 2018;138:271–81. https://doi.org/10.1016/j.diabres.2018.02.023.
4. Sharma SK, Thakur K, Kant R, Kalra S. Nurse-Led diabetes clinics in Southeast Asia: scope, feasibility, challenges and facilitators. J Diabetes Metab Disord Control. 2020;7:47–51.
5. Juster-Switlyk K, Smith AG. Updates in diabetic peripheral neuropathy. F1000Res. 2016;5:F1000 Faculty Rev-738. https://doi.org/10.12688/f1000research.7898.1.
6. Tseng KY, Wang HC, Wang YH, Su MP, Cheng KF, Cheng KI, Chang LL. Peripheral nerve denervation in streptozotocin-induced diabetic rats is reduced by cilostazol. Medicine (Kaunas, Lithuania). 2023;59(3):553. https://doi.org/10.3390/medicina59030553.
7. Hicks CW, Selvin E. Epidemiology of peripheral neuropathy and lower extremity disease in diabetes. Curr Diabetes Rep. 2019;19(10):86. https://doi.org/10.1007/s11892-019-1212-8.
8. Zhang P, Lu J, Jing Y, Tang S, Zhu D, Bi Y. Global epidemiology of diabetic foot ulceration: a systematic review and meta-analysis. Ann Med. 2017;49(2):106–16. https://doi.org/10.1080/07853890.2016.1231932.
9. Pop RB, Ang L, Boulton AJM. Diagnosis and treatment of painful diabetic peripheral neuropathy. American Diabetes Association; 2022.
10. Lu Y, Xing P, Cai X, Luo D, Li R, et al. Prevalence and risk factors for diabetic peripheral neuropathy in type 2 diabetic patients from 14 countries: estimates of the INTERPRET-DD study. Front Public Health. 2020;8:534372. https://doi.org/10.3389/fpubh.2020.534372.
11. Iqbal Z, Azmi S, Yadav R, Ferdousi M, Kumar M, Cuthbertson DJ, et al. Diabetic peripheral neuropathy: epidemiology, diagnosis, and pharmacotherapy. Clin Ther. 2018;40(6):828–49. https://doi.org/10.1016/j.clinthera.2018.04.001.
12. Chang MC, Yang S. Diabetic peripheral neuropathy essentials: a narrative review. Ann Palliat Med. 2023;12(2):390–8. https://doi.org/10.21037/apm-22-693.
13. Dinh Le T, Phi Thi Nguyen N, Thanh Thi Tran H, Luong Cong T, et al. Diabetic peripheral neuropathy associated with cardiovascular risk factors and glucagon-like peptide-1 concentrations among newly diagnosed patients with type 2 diabetes mellitus. Diabetes Metab Syndr Obes. 2022;15:35–44. https://doi.org/10.2147/DMSO.S344532.
14. Andersen ST, Witte DR, Dalsgaard EM, Andersen H, Nawroth P, et al. Risk factors for incident diabetic polyneuropathy in a cohort with screen-detected type 2 diabetes followed for 13 years: ADDITION-Denmark. Diabetes Care. 2018;41(5):1068–75. https://doi.org/10.2337/dc17-2062.
15. Hu Hanquan A, Teo Li Wen M. Prevalence of diabetic peripheral neuropathy in patients with type 2 diabetes mellitus at a tertiary referral center in Singapore. Proc Singap Healthc. 2020;30:265–70.
16. Callaghan BC, Gao L, Li Y, Zhou X, Reynolds E, Banerjee M, et al. Diabetes and obesity are the main metabolic drivers of peripheral neuropathy. Ann Clin Transl Neurol. 2018;5(4):397–405. https://doi.org/10.1002/acn3.531.
17. Zhang H, Vladimir C, Zhang Z, Zhou W, Xu J, Zhao W, et al. Serum uric acid levels are related to diabetic peripheral neuropathy, especially for motor conduction velocity of tibial nerve in type 2 diabetes mellitus patients. J Diabetes Res. 2023;2023:3060013. https://doi.org/10.1155/2023/3060013.
18. Feldman EL, Nave KA, Jensen TS, Bennett DLH. New horizons in diabetic neuropathy: mechanisms, bioenergetics, and pain. Neuron. 2017;93(6):1296–313. https://doi.org/10.1016/j.neuron.2017.02.005.

19. Zhang Y, Zhang S, Pan L, Wang B, Sun Y, Gao L, et al. Painful Diabetic Peripheral Neuropathy Study of Chinese Outpatients (PDNSCOPE): a multicentre cross-sectional registry study of clinical characteristics and treatment in Mainland China. Pain Ther. 2021;10(2):1355–73. https://doi.org/10.1007/s40122-021-00281-w.
20. Stino AM, Smith AG. Peripheral neuropathy in prediabetes and the metabolic syndrome. J Diabetes Investig. 2017;8(5):646–55. https://doi.org/10.1111/jdi.12650.
21. Feldman EL, Callaghan BC, Pop-Busui R, Zochodne DW, et al. Diabetic neuropathy. Nat Rev Dis Primers. 2019;5(1):42. https://doi.org/10.1038/s41572-019-0097-9.
22. Bodman MA, Varacallo M. Peripheral diabetic neuropathy. In: StatPearls. StatPearls Publishing; 2023.
23. Schreiber AK, Nones CF, Reis RC, Chichorro JG, Cunha JM. Diabetic neuropathic pain: physiopathology and treatment. World J Diabetes. 2015;6(3):432–44. https://doi.org/10.4239/wjd.v6.i3.432.
24. Rossboth S, Rossboth B, Schoenherr H, Lechleitner M, Oberaigner W. Risk factors for diabetic foot complications among patients with type 2 diabetes in Austria—a registry-based retrospective cohort study. Endocrinol Diabetes Metab. 2021;4(4):e00286. https://doi.org/10.1002/edm2.286.
25. Román-Pintos LM, Villegas-Rivera G, Rodríguez-Carrizalez AD, Miranda-Díaz AG, Cardona-Muñoz EG. Diabetic polyneuropathy in type 2 diabetes mellitus: inflammation, oxidative stress, and mitochondrial function. J Diabetes Res. 2016;2016:3425617. https://doi.org/10.1155/2016/3425617.
26. Ristikj-Stomnaroska D, Risteska-Nejashmikj V, Papazova M. Role of inflammation in the pathogenesis of diabetic peripheral neuropathy. Open Access Maced J Med Sci. 2019;7(14):2267–70. https://doi.org/10.3889/oamjms.2019.646.
27. Gonçalves NP, Vægter CB, Andersen H, Østergaard L, Calcutt NA, Jensen TS. Schwann cell interactions with axons and microvessels in diabetic neuropathy. Nat Rev Neurol. 2017;13(3):135–47. https://doi.org/10.1038/nrneurol.2016.201.
28. Cheng C, Kobayashi M, Martinez JA, Ng H, et al. Evidence for epigenetic regulation of gene expression and function in chronic experimental diabetic neuropathy. J Neuropathol Exp Neurol. 2015;74(8):804–17. https://doi.org/10.1097/NEN.0000000000000219.
29. Barrett EJ, Liu Z, Khamaisi M, King GL, Klein R, et al. Diabetic microvascular disease: an endocrine society scientific statement. J Clin Endocrinol Metab. 2017;102(12):4343–410. https://doi.org/10.1210/jc.2017-01922.
30. Thomas PK. Classification, differential diagnosis, and staging of diabetic peripheral neuropathy. Diabetes. 1997;46(2):S54–7. https://doi.org/10.2337/diab.46.2.s54.
31. Pop-Busui R, Boulton AJ, Feldman EL, Bril V, Freeman R, et al. Diabetic neuropathy: a position statement by the American Diabetes Association. Diabetes Care. 2017;40(1):136–54. https://doi.org/10.2337/dc16-2042.
32. Amin N, Doupis J. Diabetic foot disease: from the evaluation of the "foot at risk" to the novel diabetic ulcer treatment modalities. World J Diabetes. 2016;7(7):153–64.
33. Abraham M, Sudan HH, Pavithra V. Diabetic peripheral neuropathy. IntechOpen; 2022. https://doi.org/10.5772/intechopen.100859.
34. Anandhanarayanan A, Teh K, Goonoo M, et al. Diabetic neuropathies. 2022. Available from: https://www.ncbi.nlm.nih.gov/books/NBK279175/..
35. Yang Z, Zhang Y, Chen R, Huang Y, Ji L, Sun F, Hong T, Zhan S. Simple tests to screen for diabetic peripheral neuropathy. Cochrane Database Syst Rev. 2018;7:CD010975. https://doi.org/10.1002/14651858.CD010975.pub2.
36. Bajwa H, Al KY. Physiology, vibratory sense. StatPearls Publishing; 2024. Available from: https://www.ncbi.nlm.nih.gov/books/NBK542288/
37. Kirthi V, Perumbalath A, Brown E, Nevitt S, Petropoulos IN, et al. Prevalence of peripheral neuropathy in pre-diabetes: a systematic review. BMJ Open Diabetes Res Care. 2021;9(1):e002040. https://doi.org/10.1136/bmjdrc-2020-002040.
38. Pfannkuche A, Alhajjar A, Ming A, Walter I, et al. Prevalence and risk factors of diabetic peripheral neuropathy in a diabetics cohort: register initiative "diabetes and nerves". Endocrine Metab Sci. 2020;1(2):100053.

39. Cg SK, Maiya AG, Hande HM, Vidyasagar S, Rao K, Rajagopal KV. Efficacy of low-level laser therapy on painful diabetic peripheral neuropathy. Laser Ther. 2015;24(3):195–200. https://doi.org/10.5978/islsm.15-OR-12.
40. Monteiro RL, Ferreira JSSP, Silva ÉQ, Donini A, Cruvinel-Júnior RH, Verissímo JL, et al. Feasibility and preliminary efficacy of a foot-ankle exercise program aiming to improve foot-ankle functionality and gait biomechanics in people with diabetic neuropathy: a randomized controlled trial. Sensors. 2020;20:5129. https://doi.org/10.3390/s20185129.
41. Rahbar S, Naimi SS, Soltani AR, Rahimi A, Baghban AA, Rashedi V, Tavakkoli H. Improvement in biochemical parameters in patients with type 2 diabetes after twenty-four sessions of aerobic exercise: a randomized controlled trial. Iranian Red Crescent Med J. 2017;19(7):e13931. https://doi.org/10.5812/ircmj.13931.
42. Jahantigh Akbari N, Hosseinifar M, Naimi SS, Mikaili S, Rahbar S. The efficacy of physiotherapy interventions in mitigating the symptoms and complications of diabetic peripheral neuropathy: a systematic review. J Diabetes Metab Disord. 2020;19(2):1995–2004. https://doi.org/10.1007/s40200-020-00652-8.
43. Kirwan JP, Sacks J, Nieuwoudt S. The essential role of exercise in the management of type 2 diabetes. Cleve Clin J Med. 2017;84(7):S15–21. https://doi.org/10.3949/ccjm.84.s1.03.
44. Wang J-S. et al. Tai Chi Chuan training to enhance microcirculatory function in healthy elderly men. Arch Phys Med Rehabil. 2011;82(9):1176–80. https://doi.org/10.1053/apmr.2001.24305.
45. Li X, Si H, Chen Y, Li S, Yin N, Wang Z. Effects of fitness qigong and tai chi on middle-aged and elderly patients with type 2 diabetes mellitus. PLoS One. 2020;15(12):e0243989. https://doi.org/10.1371/journal.pone.0243989.
46. Allet L. et al. The gait and balance of patients with diabetes can be improved: a randomised controlled trial. Diabetologia. 2009;53(3):458–66. https://doi.org/10.1007/s00125-009-1592-4.
47. Jerome A, Jeyabalan K, Keong HK, Gharote G. Effect of mobilization on ankle mobility and balance performance in diabetic patients. Biomedicine. 2019;39(2):305–9.
48. Kluding PM, Bareiss SK, Hastings M, Marcus RL, Sinacore DR, Mueller MJ. Physical training and activity in people with diabetic peripheral neuropathy: paradigm shift. Phys Ther. 2017;97(1):31–43. https://doi.org/10.2522/ptj.20160124.
49. Malik R. et al. Microangiopathy in human diabetic neuropathy: relationship between capillary abnormalities and the severity of neuropathy. Diabetologia. 1989;32(2):92–102. https://doi.org/10.1007/BF00505180
50. El Hage R, Knippschild U, Arnold T, Hinterseher I. Stem cell-based therapy: a promising treatment for diabetic foot ulcer. Biomedicines. 2022;10:1507. https://doi.org/10.3390/biomedicines10071507.
51. Cameron NE. et al. Nerve function in experimental diabetes in rats: effects of electrical stimulation. Am J Physiol. 1993; 264(2 Pt 1):E161-6. https://doi.org/10.1152/ajpendo.1993.264.2.E161.
52. Mo X. et al. Effect of electro-acupuncture and transcutaneous electric nerve stimulation on experimental diabetes and its neuropathy. Zhen ci yan jiu = Acupunct Res. 1996;21(3):55–9.
53. Cui H, Yu H, Huang X, Wu L, Zhong W, Gou Y, Cao X, Liu Y, Hong Y, Zhang S, Zhan M, Li G, Yang Z. Electroacupuncture and transcutaneous electrical nerve stimulation induced sensations in Bell's Palsy patients: a quantitative current intensity analysis. Front Neurosci. 2021;15:692088. https://doi.org/10.3389/fnins.2021.692088.
54. Ahmed S, Barwick A, Butterworth P, Nancarrow S. Footwear and insole design features that reduce neuropathic plantar forefoot ulcer risk in people with diabetes: a systematic literature review. J Foot Ankle Res. 2020;13(1):30. https://doi.org/10.1186/s13047-020-00400-4.

Chapter 2
Assessment and Diagnostic Methods to Evaluate Diabetic Peripheral Neuropathy

Nidhi Sharma and Simranjeet Kaur

Contents

2.1 Introduction

Diabetic peripheral neuropathy (DPN) is a prevalent and debilitating complication of diabetes mellitus that significantly impacts the lives of millions of individuals worldwide [1]. As a prevalent type of neuropathy, DPN develops due to extended periods of elevated blood sugar levels, leading to damage in the peripheral nervous system. This condition presents a complex and multifaceted challenge, affecting sensory, motor, and autonomic nerve fibers, ultimately resulting in a wide range of

N. Sharma (✉) · S. Kaur
Maharishi Markandeshwar Institute of Physiotherapy and Rehabilitation, Maharishi Markandeshwar (Deemed to be University), Ambala, Haryana, India
e-mail: sharma.nidhi.physio@mmumullana.org; dr.simranjeet.kaur@mmumullana.org

© The Author(s), under exclusive license to Springer Nature Singapore Pte Ltd. 2024

M. Goyal, K. Goyal (eds.), *Rehabilitation in Diabetic Peripheral Neuropathy*,
https://doi.org/10.1007/978-981-97-9290-0_2

distressing symptoms and functional impairments [2]. Evaluating DPN is crucial for identifying it at an early stage, effective management, and prevention of potential complications [3]. This introduction will delve into the significance of assessing DPN, highlighting the methods, tools, and clinical approaches that healthcare professionals employ to diagnose and monitor this condition, aiming to improve patients' quality of life and mitigate the long-term consequences of DPN.

2.2 Assessment and Identification of Diabetic Neuropathy

The assessment and identification of diabetic neuropathy (DPN) require a comprehensive evaluation involving various clinical, neurological, and electrophysiological methods. Early detection is crucial to prevent the advancement of the condition and to initiate appropriate management. Below, we'll explore the assessment procedure and diagnosis of DPN in detail.

2.2.1 Clinical Evaluation

2.2.1.1 Medical History

This step involves obtaining a comprehensive medical history from the patient. It includes information about the duration of diabetes, glycemic control, and any family history of neuropathy. Additionally, any relevant comorbidities, such as vascular disease or kidney problems, should be explored [4, 5].

2.2.1.2 Symptom Assessment

Patients with DPN often experience a range of symptoms. These can include numbness, tingling, burning sensations, or pain in the extremities, particularly in the feet and legs. Motor symptoms like muscle weakness and atrophy may also be present. The type and severity of these symptoms are crucial for diagnosis [6].

2.2.2 Clinical Examination

2.2.2.1 Neurological Examination

A thorough neurological examination by a healthcare professional is vital. This assessment evaluates sensory and motor functions. It may include testing reflexes, assessing muscle strength, coordination, and sensory perception. For example, a pinprick test may be performed to assess pain perception, while the ability to detect vibrations can be checked using a tuning fork [7].

2.2.2.2 Vascular Assessment

Impaired blood circulation can contribute to neuropathic symptoms. A vascular assessment is important to ensure that reduced blood flow is not exacerbating the neuropathy. Checking for pedal pulses and skin temperature is a part of this assessment [1].

2.2.3 Objective Testing (Fig. 2.1)

2.2.3.1 Monofilament Testing [1, 4, 8, 9]

Testing by monofilament is a straightforward and commonly employed technique for evaluating peripheral neuropathy, particularly in the context of diabetes. A single filament has been used for this test, which is a thin, flexible filament that can be applied to specific points on the skin to assess tactile sensation. The commonest application of monofilament testing is in evaluating DPN, a complication of diabetes characterized by nerve damage in the extremities.

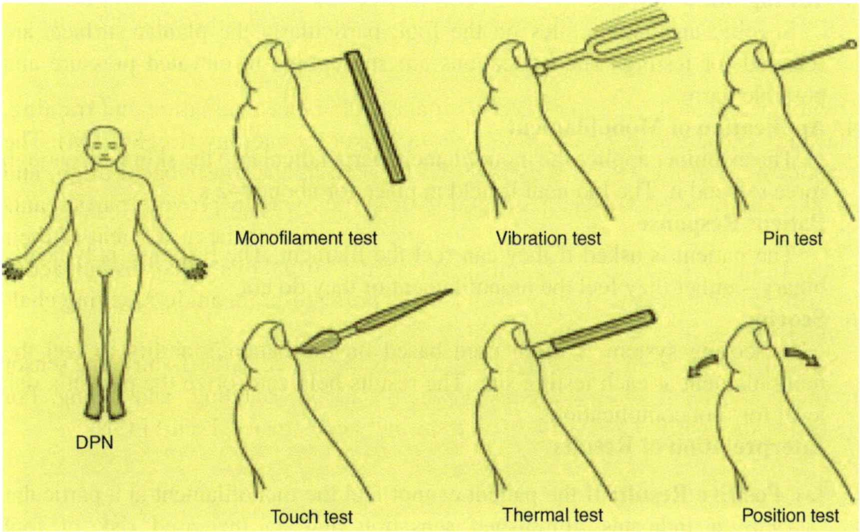

Fig. 2.1 Assessment tools for diabetic peripheral neuropathy (DPN) include bedside tests for both large fiber (10-g monofilament, 128-Hz tuning fork, touch, and joint position) and small fiber function (cold and warm sensation, pinprick) [12]

2.2.3.1.1 Purpose of Monofilament Testing

1. **Detection of Peripheral Neuropathy**
   The primary purpose of monofilament testing is to detect the loss of protective sensation in the feet and lower extremities. This is crucial in diabetes, where peripheral neuropathy can lead to reduced sensation, increasing the risk of foot injuries and complications.
2. **Risk Assessment**
   Monofilament testing helps assess the risk of foot ulceration and lower extremity amputation in individuals with diabetes. Those who have diminished sensation are at a higher risk of injuries going unnoticed, leading to complications.

2.2.3.1.2 Procedure

1. **Monofilament Selection**
   Monofilaments are typically made of nylon or similar materials. They come in different thicknesses, and a standard set of monofilaments with varying forces is often used. The most commonly used monofilament for clinical testing applies a force equivalent to 10 g of pressure.
2. **Patient Positioning**
   The patient is usually in a seated or supine position. It's essential to ensure a quiet and distraction-free environment for accurate testing.
3. **Testing Sites**
   Specific anatomical sites on the foot, particularly the plantar surface, are selected for testing. These locations are susceptible to elevated pressure and possible harm.
4. **Application of Monofilament**
   The examiner applies the monofilament perpendicular to the skin with enough force to bend it. The filament is held in place for about 1–2 s.
5. **Patient Response**
   The patient is asked if they can feel the filament. The response is typically binary—either they feel the monofilament or they do not.
6. **Scoring**
   A scoring system is often used based on the patient's ability to feel the monofilament at each testing site. The results help categorize the patient's risk level for foot complications.
7. **Interpretation of Results**

   (a) **Positive Result:** If the patient cannot feel the monofilament at a particular site, it indicates diminished sensation and an increased risk of foot complications.

(b) **Negative Result:** If the patient can feel the monofilament at all tested sites, it suggests intact protective sensation.

2.2.3.1.3 Considerations

1. **Standardization**
   To ensure consistency and reliability, monofilament testing should be performed using standardized protocols, including the selection of appropriate monofilaments and testing sites.
2. **Complementary Assessments**
   Monofilament testing is frequently utilized alongside additional evaluations, such as vibration perception testing and ankle reflex assessments, for a more comprehensive evaluation of neuropathy.
3. **Regular Monitoring**
   Periodic monofilament testing is recommended for individuals at risk of neuropathy, especially those with diabetes. Consistent monitoring aids in identifying alterations in sensation over time.

   Monofilament testing is a valuable and cost-effective tool in the clinical assessment of peripheral neuropathy, particularly in the diabetic population. It provides a quick and reliable means of identifying individuals at risk of foot complications, allowing for timely interventions to prevent serious complications such as ulcers and amputations.

2.2.3.2 Vibration Perception Threshold (VPT) [1, 4, 8–10]

Vibration perception threshold (VPT) testing is a diagnostic method used to assess peripheral neuropathy, particularly in the context of conditions such as diabetes. It measures a person's ability to perceive vibratory stimuli, which is an important aspect of sensory function. The test is particularly relevant in detecting DPN, a common complication of diabetes characterized by nerve damage in the extremities.

2.2.3.2.1 Purpose of Vibration Perception Threshold Testing

1. **Early Detection of Neuropathy**
   VPT testing is employed to detect early signs of neuropathy, especially in individuals at risk, such as those with diabetes. Timely identification permits prompt interventions to halt the advancement of neuropathy.
2. **Assessment of Sensory Function**
   The ability to perceive vibrations is crucial for balance, coordination, and protection against injury. VPT testing provides information about sensory function in the lower extremities, where neuropathy commonly occurs.

2.2.3.2.2 Procedure

1. **Equipment**
   VPT testing is often performed using a handheld device called a vibrometer or a biothesiometer. This device produces controlled vibrations that are applied to specific sites on the skin.
2. **Patient Positioning**
   The patient is usually seated or lying down in a comfortable position. It's important to ensure a quiet and distraction-free environment for accurate testing.
3. **Testing Sites**
   Common testing sites include the bony prominences on the feet, particularly the great toe or the metatarsal heads. These locations are selected due to their susceptibility to high pressure and are often affected in peripheral neuropathy.
4. **Application of Vibratory Stimulus**
   The examiner applies the vibrating probe to the chosen testing site. The vibration's strength is incrementally raised to the threshold where the patient indicates they can perceive it.
5. **Patient Response**
   The response of the patient was recorded as the moment, and the vibration was felt by the patient. This threshold level is recorded as the VPT.

2.2.3.2.3 Interpretation of Results

(a) **Increased VPT**: An increased VPT indicates a reduced ability to perceive vibrations, suggesting sensory nerve dysfunction. This is often seen in conditions such as diabetic neuropathy.
(b) **Normal VPT**: A normal VPT suggests intact sensory function at the tested sites.

2.2.3.2.4 Considerations

1. **Standardization**
   To ensure consistency and reliability, VPT testing should be performed using standardized protocols, including the selection of appropriate testing sites and the calibration of the vibrometer.
2. **Complementary Assessments**
   VPT testing is usually performed along with different sensory tests, such as monofilament testing and ankle reflex assessments, for a more comprehensive evaluation of neuropathy.
3. **Risk Assessment**
   Elevated VPT levels correlate with a heightened likelihood of foot complications, such as ulcers and amputations. Regular monitoring helps track changes in sensory function over time.

Assessing VPT is an invaluable tool in the evaluation of peripheral neuropathy clinically, providing quantitative information about sensory function in the lower extremities. VPT testing holds particular significance in the early detection of neuropathy, affording opportunities for prompt interventions to mitigate complications. When integrated with complementary sensory evaluations, such as monofilament testing and nerve conduction studies, VPT assessment enhances the comprehensive appraisal of peripheral neuropathy. This integrative approach enables healthcare practitioners to formulate tailored therapeutic regimens tailored to the individual needs of patients at risk of neuropathic conditions.

2.2.3.3 Temperature Sensitivity Testing [2, 4, 7, 11]

Temperature sensitivity testing, also known as thermal perception testing, is a diagnostic method used to assess the sensory function of peripheral nerves, especially in the context of neuropathic conditions such as DPN. This type of testing evaluates a person's ability to detect and discriminate between different temperatures, which is crucial for protective responses and overall sensory function.

2.2.3.3.1 Purpose of Temperature Sensitivity Testing

1. **Assessment of Small Fiber Neuropathy**:
   Small neurons are accountable for temperature sensation. Temperature sensitivity testing helps in evaluating small fiber neuropathy, which is usually linked with diabetes and other neuropathic disorders.
2. **Detection in the initial stages of Neuropathy:**
   Similar to other sensory tests, temperature sensitivity testing is employed for the identification of neuropathy during the initial stages, permitting prompt action and prevention of complications.

2.2.3.3.2 Procedure

1. **Equipment:**
   Examinations can be conducted utilizing diverse techniques, such as thermal stimulators, thermal rollers, or thermodes. These devices allow for the controlled application of warm and cold stimuli.
2. **Patient Positioning:**
   The patient is typically seated comfortably. It's important to ensure that the testing environment is free from drafts or other factors that could affect temperature perception.
3. **Testing Sites:**

Common testing sites include the dorsum (top) and plantar (bottom) surfaces of the foot which are often affected in peripheral neuropathy and are crucial for protective sensation.

4. **Application of Thermal Stimuli:**
   The examiner applies controlled warm or cold stimuli to the selected testing sites. The temperature range may vary, but it often includes warm (e.g., 40 °C) and cold (e.g., 5 °C) temperatures.
5. **Patient Response:**
   The patient is requested to communicate when they initially sense the temperature alteration, and when the sensation becomes painful or uncomfortable. This helps assess both warm and cold detection thresholds.
6. **Quantitative Assessment:**
   Some methods of temperature sensitivity testing provide quantitative data, allowing for the measurement of specific thresholds, such as the temperature at which the patient first perceives the stimulus.

2.2.3.3.3 Interpretation of Results

(a) **Increased Detection Thresholds:** Elevated detection thresholds for warm or cold stimuli suggest reduced sensitivity and may indicate sensory nerve dysfunction, as seen in neuropathic conditions like DPN.
(b) **Painful Sensations at Higher Temperatures:** If the patient reports pain or discomfort at higher temperatures than expected, it may indicate thermal hyperalgesia, a heightened sensitivity to temperature stimuli often associated with neuropathy.

2.2.3.3.4 Considerations

1. **Standardization:**
   To ensure reliability, temperature sensitivity testing should be performed using standardized protocols, including the selection of appropriate testing sites and the calibration of the equipment.
2. **Complementary Assessments:**
   Temperature sensitivity testing is often used alongside other sensory tests, such as VPT and monofilament testing, for the in-depth assessment of neuropathy.
3. **Patient Variability:**
   Demographic variables and individual physiological variations can exert influence on temperature perception. Clinicians must meticulously consider these factors during the interpretation of test findings.

Temperature sensitivity testing is a worthwhile component of the clinical assessment of DPN, offering understanding into the operation of small nerve fibers responsible for sensing temperature. When combined with other sensory tests, it contributes to a comprehensive evaluation of neuropathy, aiding healthcare providers in diagnosing and managing conditions that affect sensory function in the extremities. Early detection through temperature sensitivity testing allows for proactive interventions to prevent complications associated with peripheral neuropathy.

2.2.3.4 Nerve Conduction Studies (NCS) [1, 4, 6, 8, 11, 13]

Nerve conduction studies (NCS) are electro-diagnostic tests that assess the function and integrity of peripheral nerves, used in the diagnosis and evaluation of DPN. DPN, a consequence of diabetes, occurs due to nerve impairment in the limbs due to prolonged exposure to high blood glucose levels. Nerve conduction studies are essential for accurately assessing the level and seriousness of nerve impairment in diabetes patients.

2.2.3.4.1 Purpose of Nerve Conduction Studies in DPN

1. **Objective Assessment:** Nerve conduction studies provide an objective and quantitative assessment of the function of peripheral nerves. This holds significance in assessing the degree of nerve injury in DPN.
2. **Differential Diagnosis:** Nerve conduction studies aid in distinguishing between various forms of neuropathy, eliminating alternative reasons for nerve malfunction.
3. **Localization of Nerve Damage:** NCS can help determine the location of nerve damage, whether it's in the sensory or motor nerves, and identify the specific nerves affected.
4. **Severity Grading:** The outcome of NCS can be used to grade the extent of neuropathy, ranging from mild to severe.

2.2.3.4.2 Procedure

1. **Electrode Placement:** On the skin covering the nerves that are being examined, electrodes are applied. Surface electrodes are typically employed, and they are positioned at particular locations throughout the nerve pathway.
2. **Stimulation of Nerves:** The nerves are stimulated with a small electric impulse, and the resulting electrical activity is recorded. In research on motor nerve conduction, a motor nerve is stimulated, whereas in studies on sensory nerve conduction, a sensory nerve is stimulated.
3. **Measurement of Nerve Conduction Velocity:** One of the key parameters measured is nerve conduction velocity, which is the speed at which the electrical impulse travels along the nerve. Slowed conduction velocity is a common finding in diabetic neuropathy.

4. **Amplitude Measurements:** The amplitude of the recorded electrical response is also measured. Reduced amplitude may indicate axonal damage or demyelination.
5. **F-Wave and H-Reflex Studies:** F-waves (motor nerve) and H-reflexes (sensory nerve) may be studied. These reactions furnish supplementary details regarding the condition of nerve routes.
6. **Temperature Control:** The temperature of the testing room and the patient's extremities is controlled because temperature can affect nerve conduction.

2.2.3.4.3 Interpretation of Results: (Fig. 2.2) [14–17]

(a) **Reduced Nerve Conduction Velocity:** Slowed nerve conduction velocity is a characteristic finding in diabetic neuropathy and is indicative of damage to the myelin sheath or the axon.
(b) **Reduced Amplitude:** Reduced amplitude of the recorded response may suggest axonal loss or demyelination.
(c) **Prolonged Latency:** Prolonged latency of F-waves or H-reflexes may indicate abnormalities in nerve transmission.
(d) **Side-to-Side Comparison:** Asymmetry of nerve involvement can be better understood by comparing the afflicted and unaffected sides.

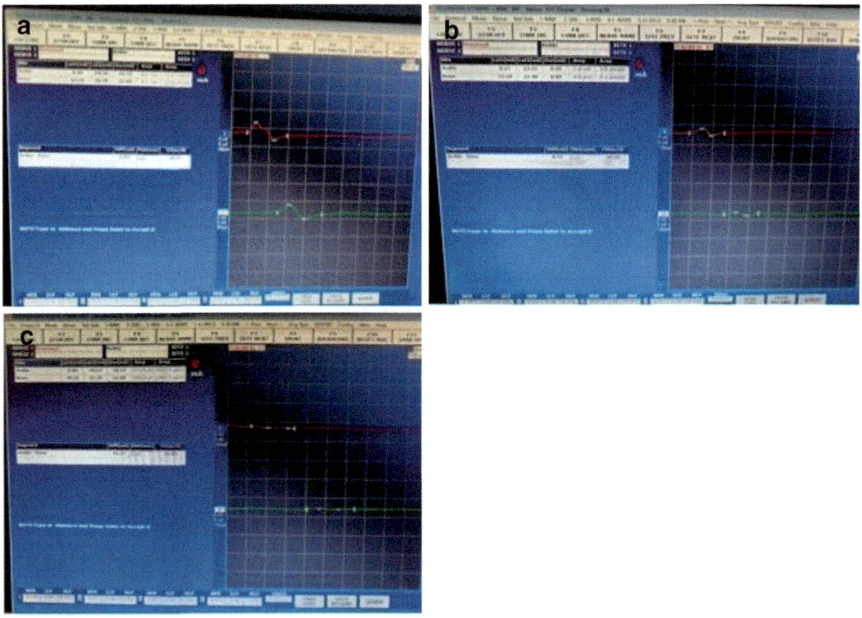

Fig. 2.2 Graphical representation of peroneal nerve activity in normal state (**a**), moderately affected (**b**), and severely affected (**c**) [15, 17]

Table 2.1 Typical values for lower extremity nerve conduction studies of adults

S. No.	Nerve	Record	Amplitude (mV)	Conduction velocity (m/s)	Distal latency (ms)	Distal distance (cm)	Minimal F latency (ms)	Minimal H latency (ms)
1.	Peroneal	Extensor Digitorum Brevis (EDB)	≥2.0	44	≤6.5	9	≤56	N/A
2.	Peroneal[a]	Tibialis anterior (TA)	≥3.0	41	≤6.7	5–10	–	–
3.	Tibial	Abductor Hallucis Longus (EHL)	≥4.0	41	≤5.8	9	≤56	≤34[b]
4.	Tibial[a]	Abductor Digiti Quinti Pedis	≥3.0	41	≤6.3	Variable	–	–

[a]In cases of asymmetrical symptoms, comparing amplitudes between sides is more helpful than referencing normal values
[b]Compare side by side, and any latency difference exceeding 1.5 ms between sides is considered abnormal

Table 2.1 represents typical values for lower extremity nerve conduction studies of adults [14–16].

2.2.3.4.4 Considerations

1. **Clinical Correlation:** When nerve conduction investigations are combined with other diagnostic findings and the patient's clinical complaints, they provide the most useful information.
2. **Other Tests:** Frequently, NCS is utilized in combination with additional examinations, like electromyography (EMG), to offer a thorough evaluation of nerve and muscle performance.
3. **Serial Testing:** Consecutive nerve conduction studies conducted over a period can aid in tracking the advancement of neuropathy and the efficacy of treatments.

While tests for nerve conduction are essential for identifying and assessing DPN, they are also often used in conjunction with other clinical and laboratory assessments to provide a comprehensive understanding of diabetic neuropathy. Nerve conduction studies provide factual insights into the degree and severity of nerve impairment, which aids medical professionals in developing accurate diagnoses and treatment plans.

2.2.3.5 Electromyography (EMG) [1, 4, 6, 8, 11, 13]

Electromyography (EMG) assesses the electrical activity of muscles. It can help determine if muscle weakness is due to nerve damage or other causes. Interpreting EMG results in the context of DPN involves assessing the electrical activity of muscles and the function of peripheral nerves.

2.2.3.5.1 EMG Results and Their Implications for DPN

1. **Spontaneous Activity:**
   (a) **Normal Result:** In healthy muscles, there should be no spontaneous activity (fibrillation potentials or positive sharp waves) during needle EMG when the muscle is at rest.
   (b) **Abnormal Result:** Presence of spontaneous activity may indicate denervation, which is common in DPN. This suggests that the nerves controlling the muscle are damaged, leading to abnormal electrical signals.
2. **Motor Unit Recruitment:**
   (a) **Normal Result:** During voluntary muscle contraction, there should be a normal recruitment pattern of motor units, and the muscle should generate smooth, coordinated activity.
   (b) **Abnormal Result:** In DPN, there may be reduced recruitment of motor units, leading to a decreased amplitude of the recorded electrical signals. This reflects impaired nerve-muscle communication.
3. **Motor Unit Action Potential (MUAP):**
   (a) **Normal Result**: MUAPs in healthy muscles are of normal duration and amplitude.
   (b) **Abnormal Result**: In DPN, MUAPs may show abnormal features, such as prolonged duration or reduced amplitude, indicating dysfunction in the peripheral nerves.

Table 2.2 represents the mean MUAP duration based on age and muscle group involved [17, 18].

2.2.3.5.2 Interpretation

1. **Severity of Neuropathy:** The degree and acuteness of abnormalities observed in EMG can provide insights into the degree of neuropathy. More severe neuropathy is often associated with pronounced spontaneous activity, reduced recruitment, and abnormal MUAPs.

Table 2.2 Mean MUAP duration (in ms) based on age and muscle group

S. No.	Age (in years)	Gastrocnemius	Anterior tibialis	Fibularis (Peroneus) Longus	EDB
1.	0–4	6.4–8.2	8.0–10.2	6.8–7.4	6.3–8.1
2.	5–9	6.5–8.8	8.1–11.0	5.9–7.9	6.4–8.7
3.	10–14	6.6–9.1	8.2–11.3	5.9–8.2	6.5–9.0
4.	15–19	7.0–9.9	8.7–12.3	6.3–8.9	6.9–9.8
5.	20–29	7.7–10.7	9.6–13.3	6.9–9.6	7.6–10.6
6.	30–39	9.0–12.1	11.2–15.1	8.1–10.9	8.9–12.0
7.	40–49	9.6–12.8	11.9–15.9	8.6–11.5	9.5–12.7
8.	50–59	10.4–13.6	12.9–16.9	9.4–12.2	10.3–13.5
9.	60–69	10.8–14.1	13.4–17.5	9.7–12.7	10.7–14.0
10.	70–79	11.1–14.4	13.8–17.9	10.0–13.0	11.0–14.3

EDB Extensor Digitorum Brevis

2. **Localization of Lesions**: EMG can help determine whether nerve damage is more proximal (closer to the spinal cord) or distal (farther from the spinal cord), aiding in the localization of lesions.
3. **Correlation with Clinical Findings:** It's essential to correlate EMG results with the patient's clinical symptoms and other diagnostic examinations to develop a thorough comprehension of the neuropathic state.
4. **Monitoring Progression:** Repeat EMG studies over time can help monitor the progression of neuropathy and the effectiveness of interventions.

Table 2.3 represents the MUAP patterns according to pathological lesions [17, 18].

2.2.3.5.3 Limitations and Considerations

(a) **Operator Skill:** Interpretation of EMG results requires expertise, and the results should be analyzed by a skilled neurophysiologist.
(b) **Variability:** EMG findings can vary, and a single test might not be able to fully diagnose neuropathy. It might take several tests periodically to get an accurate assessment.

EMG is a valuable tool for evaluating DPN by providing objective data on muscle and nerve function. Interpreting the results requires a combination of clinical correlation, consideration of the patient's symptoms, and expertise in neurophysiology. It plays a crucial role in the diagnosis, localization, and monitoring of DPN, helping healthcare professionals tailor treatment plans for affected individuals.

Table 2.3 MUAP patterns according to pathology

S. No.	Pathology	MUAP morphology			MUAP firing pattern	
		Duration	Amplitude	Phases	Activation	Recruitment
1.	Acute neuropathic-axonal	Typical	Typical	Typical	Typical	–
2.	Chronic neuropathic-axonal	+	+	+	Typical	–
3.	Neuropathic-Demylienating (CV slowing alone)	Typical	Typical	Typical	Typical	Typical
4.	Neuropathic-Demylienating (conduction block)	Typical	Typical	Typical	Typical	–
5.	Early reinnervation after severe denervation (nascent unit)	–	–	+	Typical	––
6.	Acute Myopathic	–	–	+	Typical	Typical/ early
7.	Chronic Myopathic	+/–	+/–	+	Typical	Typical/ early
8.	Myopathic-endsatge	+/–	+/–	+	Typical	––

MUAP Motor Unit Action Potential; + increased; – decreased; +/– may be increased or decreased; ++ marked increase; –– marked decrease

2.2.3.6 Quantitative Sensory Testing (QST) [3, 9]

Quantitative sensory testing (QST) is a non-invasive method used to assess the function of peripheral sensory nerves and evaluate sensory perception thresholds. It is particularly relevant in the context of DPN, where nerve damage can lead to alterations in sensation. QST provides quantitative measures of sensory function and can help in diagnosing and monitoring the progression of DPN.

2.2.3.6.1 Principles of Quantitative Sensory Testing

1. **Objective Measurement**: QST quantifies sensory responses to various stimuli to provide objective and standardized measurements of sensory function.
2. **Assessment of Different Modalities:** QST evaluates different sensory modalities, including touch, temperature, vibration, and pain perception, to comprehensively assess the impact of neuropathy on sensory nerves.
3. **Identification of Thresholds:** QST measures the thresholds at which individuals perceive stimuli. For example, it determines the minimum level of a stimulus (e.g., temperature or pressure) required for a person to sense it.

2.2.3.6.2 Common QST Modalities for DPN

1. **Thermal Thresholds:**
   (a) **Cold and Warm Detection Thresholds:** QST assesses the ability to perceive changes in temperature. Individuals with DPN may have altered thresholds for cold and warm sensations.
2. **Mechanical Thresholds:**
   (a) **Pressure Detection Thresholds:** Measures the pressure required for an individual to sense a stimulus.
   (b) **Vibration Detection Thresholds**: Assesses the ability to perceive vibration, which can be affected in DPN.
3. **Pain Thresholds:**
   (a) **Mechanical Pain Thresholds:** Measures the pressure at which a sensation becomes painful.
   (b) **Thermal Pain Thresholds:** Assesses the temperature at which a stimulus becomes perceived as painful.
4. **Dynamic Mechanical Allodynia:** Evaluates the perception of pain in response to normally non-painful stimuli, such as light touch or brushing.

2.2.3.6.3 Application in Diabetic Peripheral Neuropathy

1. **Early Detection:** QST has the capability to identify sensory irregularities during the initial phases of DPN, prior to the manifestation of evident clinical symptoms. This early detection is crucial for timely intervention.
2. **Monitoring Progression:** QST can be used to monitor the progression of neuropathy over time. Changes in sensory thresholds can indicate the worsening of nerve damage.
3. **Differentiation from Other Conditions:** Helps differentiate DPN from other neuropathic or non-neuropathic disorders which may have similar symptoms.
4. **Treatment Monitoring:** QST can be employed to assess the effectiveness of interventions and treatments aimed at managing DPN. Improvements in sensory thresholds may indicate a positive response to therapy.

2.2.3.6.4 Considerations and Challenges

1. **Patient Cooperation:** Patient cooperation and understanding is vital to get reliable QST results. It requires the active participation of the patient being tested.
2. **Variability:** QST results may vary between individuals, and creating standard data for particular populations is crucial for precise interpretation.

3. **Multimodal Assessment:** QST along with nerve conduction studies and clinical evaluation provides a more comprehensive assessment of DPN.

Quantitative sensory testing is a valuable tool for objectively assessing sensory function in individuals with DPN. It helps in early detection, monitoring progression, and tailoring interventions to manage the sensory symptoms associated with DPN. Combining QST with additional techniques for diagnosis helps create more focused treatment strategies and advances our understanding of how diabetes affects peripheral nerves.

2.2.3.7 Skin Biopsy [1, 2]

In cases where small fiber neuropathy is suspected, skin biopsies are used to measure intra-epidermal nerve fiber density (IENFD). A reduced IENFD is indicative of small fiber neuropathy, which is a common feature of DPN.

2.2.4 Laboratory Tests

2.2.4.1 HbA1c, or Hemoglobin A1c [7, 8, 11, 19, 20]

An individual's average level of glucose in their blood over the previous 2–3 months is determined by the HbA1c blood test. In people with diabetes mellitus, this test is frequently used to track long-term glucose control. In order to evaluate the efficacy of diabetes management techniques and lower the risk of consequences linked to raise blood sugar levels, it is imperative that healthcare practitioners together with people with diabetes have a thorough understanding of HbA1c.

2.2.4.1.1 Formation of HbA1c

HbA1c is formed through a non-enzymatic process called glycation. Blood glucose binds to hemoglobin, the oxygen-carrying protein in red blood corpuscles (RBC). This binding occurs slowly over the lifespan of RBC (which is about 2–3 months). Once formed, HbA1c remains in RBC until the cells die (typically after about 120 days).

2.2.4.1.2 Measurement and Reporting

The percentage of total hemoglobin is represented by HbA1c. The percentage reflects the proportion of hemoglobin that is glycated by glucose.

For individuals without diabetes, a normal HbA1c level is usually below 5.7%. Nevertheless, healthcare professionals frequently establish the desired range for individuals with diabetes based on their unique situations, with a common recommendation being to maintain levels below 7%.

2.2.4.1.3 Clinical Significance

1. **Long-Term Glucose Control:** HbA1c provides an average of blood glucose levels over an extended period, giving a more comprehensive picture of long-term glucose control compared to daily blood glucose monitoring.
2. **Diagnosis of Diabetes:** HbA1c levels are used as part of the diagnostic criteria for diabetes. A value of 6.5% or higher on two separate tests is often indicative of diabetes.
3. **Treatment Monitoring:** It is a key tool for healthcare providers to determine the impact of diabetes management plans and to make adjustments as needed.

2.2.4.1.4 Factors Influencing HbA1c

1. **Lifespan of Red Blood Corpuscles:** RBC count has been afflicted due to certain disorders, such as anemia or certain medical treatments, can influence HbA1c levels.
2. **Iron Deficiency:** Iron deficiency can affect HbA1c measurement and lead to inaccurate results.
3. **Ethnicity:** Certain research indicates potential variations in HbA1c levels across diverse ethnic populations.

2.2.4.1.5 Limitations

1. **Short-Term Changes:** Although HbA1c provides an average representation of level of glucose in the blood over several months, it does not account for short-term fluctuations. Daily blood glucose monitoring is essential for understanding daily variations.
2. **Individual Variation:** The relationship between HbA1c and average level of glucose in the blood can be different among different individuals. Some individuals have elevated or lower HbA1c levels for a given average blood glucose.

2.2.4.1.6 Goal Setting

Target Ranges: The recommended HbA1c targets are typically personalized according to factors such as demographic characteristics, general health, and coexisting medical conditions. A common objective for individuals with diabetes is to maintain their HbA1c levels below 7%.

2.2.4.1.7 Interpretation of Results

(a) **Well-Controlled Diabetes:** Level of HbA1c under the desired range indicates good long-term glucose control and a reduced risk of diabetes-related complications.
(b) **Poorly Controlled Diabetes:** Elevated HbA1c levels suggest poor glucose control, increasing the risk of complications.

2.2.4.1.8 Frequency of Testing

For individuals with stable blood glucose control, HbA1c is often tested every 3–6 months. When there are concerns about glucose control or at times when treatment is being adjusted, more regular testing may be advised.

HbA1c is a critical tool for assessing long-term glucose control in individuals with diabetes. Regular monitoring helps guide treatment decisions and contributes to the overall management of diabetes, minimizing the likelihood of complications brought on by high blood sugar. Diabetes patients must collaborate closely with their medical professionals to establish individualized goals and create plans of action in order to reach and maintain target HbA1c levels.

2.2.4.2 Other Laboratory Examinations [2, 4]

1. **Complete Blood Count (CBC)**
   This is done to exclude further prospective causes of neuropathy, such as anemia.
2. **Vitamin B12 Levels**
   A deficiency in vitamin B12 can cause neuropathic symptoms. It is essential to check vitamin B12 levels, as supplementation may be necessary.
3. **Thyroid Tests**
   Disorders of thyroid gland can mimic neuropathic symptoms, and it's important to rule out thyroid dysfunction.
4. **Renal Function Tests**
   Kidney disease is a common complication of diabetes and can contribute to neuropathy. Assessing renal function helps identify any kidney-related factors contributing to neuropathy.

2.2.5 Imaging Techniques [5]

2.2.5.1 Magnetic Resonance Imaging (MRI)

MRI can be utilized when there are uncertainties of nerve compression or structural abnormalities. It is particularly useful when there is uncertainty about the cause of neuropathic symptoms.

2.2.5.2 Ultrasound

High-resolution ultrasound can assess nerve morphology. This is especially helpful in assessing structural problems and entrapment of nerves.

2.2.6 Assessment of Comorbidities

As individuals with DPN are often at risk for other diabetes-related complications, including retinopathy, nephropathy, and cardiovascular disease, a comprehensive assessment of these comorbidities may be necessary. This all-encompassing method guarantees that the assessment and treatment of DPN take into account every facet of the patient's health.

2.2.7 Patient-Reported Outcomes

Patient-reported outcomes are a valuable aspect of the assessment. Patients may complete questionnaires that assess the effect of neuropathy on their quality of life. The Neuropathy Total Symptom Score (NTSS-6) and the Neuropathy Impairment Score—Lower Limb (NIS-LL) are commonly used tools to assess the severity of neuropathy and its effects on daily functioning.

2.2.7.1 Neuropathy Total Symptom Score (NTSS-6) [21, 22]

The Neuropathy Total Symptom Score (NTSS-6) is a clinical tool used to assess the severity and impact of symptoms in individuals with peripheral neuropathy. Peripheral neuropathy refers to damage or dysfunction of the peripheral nerves, which are nerves outside the brain and spinal cord. There are several possible reasons of this illness, such as diabetes, autoimmune disorders, infections, and certain medications.

The NTSS-6 is a questionnaire designed to evaluate the intensity and frequency of symptoms experienced by patients with peripheral neuropathy. It consists of six domains, each focusing on specific aspects of neuropathic symptoms. The six domains include:

1. **Pain:** This domain assesses the presence, intensity, and characteristics of pain experienced by the individual. It may include descriptors such as burning, tingling, stabbing, or electric shock-like sensations.
2. **Motor Symptoms:** Motor symptoms involve issues with movement and muscle control. The NTSS-6 evaluates weakness, cramping, and difficulties with coordination or balance.
3. **Autonomic Symptoms:** Rate at which the heart beats, pressure across the blood vessels, and digestion are examples of involuntary body functions that are

regulated by the nervous system that controls autonomic functions. This domain assesses symptoms related to autonomic dysfunction, such as changes in sweating, heart rate, or blood pressure.
4. **Vibration Sensation:** Vibration sensation is an important aspect of sensory function. This domain evaluates the individual's ability to perceive vibrations, which can be impaired in peripheral neuropathy.
5. **Hypoesthesia (Reduced Sensation):** Reduced sensation or hypoesthesia is a typical feature of neuropathy in the peripheral limbs. This domain assesses the individual's ability to perceive light touch or pressure.
6. **Sleep Disturbances:** Sleep quality can be considerably adversely affected by peripheral nerve disease. Sleep abnormalities linked to neuropathic symptoms are examined in this domain, both in terms of their frequency and intensity.

Each domain is scored individually, and the total score is calculated by summing the scores from all six domains. The NTSS-6 provides a comprehensive assessment of the impact of neuropathic symptoms on various aspects of a patient's life.

Healthcare professionals use the NTSS-6 to monitor changes in symptoms over time, assess treatment effectiveness, and tailor interventions to address specific symptom domains. It serves as a valuable tool clinically as well as for research studies focused on peripheral neuropathy. Keep in mind that while the NTSS-6 is a widely used tool, there may be variations in how it is administered and interpreted in different clinical settings. For precise and customized assessments, always seek the advice of medical experts.

2.2.7.2 The Neuropathy Impairment Score—Lower Limb (NIS-LL) [22]

Neuropathy Impairment Score—Lower Limb (NIS-LL) is a clinical assessment tool specifically designed to evaluate lower limb function in individuals with peripheral neuropathy. Peripheral neuropathy refers to damage or dysfunction of the peripheral nerves, which are nerves outside the brain and spinal cord. Numerous conditions, including diabetes, autoimmune diseases, infections, and some drugs, can cause this illness.

The NIS-LL is frequently used to measure the degree of lower limb neuropathy-related deficits in clinical trials and research investigations. It provides a standardized and systematic way to assess various aspects of sensory and motor function. The assessment is typically performed by a trained healthcare professional, such as a neurologist.

The NIS-LL includes several components, each targeting specific aspects of lower limb function:

1. **Muscle Weakness:** The examiner uses standardized testing protocols to assess the strength of the muscles in particular lower limb muscle groups. This involves testing the strength of the plantar flexors, knee extensors, knee flexors, and ankle dorsiflexors.

2. **Sensory Function:** To evaluate a person's capacity to perceive stimuli in various lower limb regions, sensory testing is done. Testing for a gentle touch, pinprick, vibration, and location sensing may be part of this.
3. **Reflexes:** Reflexes are examined to assess the integrity of the neurological pathways. Common reflexes checked in the lower limbs include the Achilles reflex (ankle jerk) and the patellar reflex (knee jerk).
4. **Nerve Conduction Studies:** While not included in the NIS-LL score, nerve conduction studies may be performed alongside the clinical assessment to provide objective data on nerve function. These studies involve measuring the speed and amplitude of nerve impulses as they travel along peripheral nerves.

Higher scores indicate more severe impairment. The NIS-LL is assessed on a preset scale for each component. The total NIS-LL score is then calculated by summing the individual scores from each component. This cumulative score provides an overall measure of the severity of neuropathy-related impairments in the lower limbs.

The NIS-LL is particularly valuable in clinical trials and research settings, where standard tests are essential for evaluating treatment outcomes and disease progression. It helps healthcare professionals and researchers track changes in neuropathy-related impairments over time, assess treatment efficacy, and compare outcomes have been compared between several patient groups.

It's crucial to remember that the NIS-LL is only one instrument for evaluating peripheral neuropathy, and that its application may change depending on the clinical and research context. Always seek the advice of medical professionals to ensure precise and customized assessments.

2.2.8 Multidisciplinary Approach

A multidisciplinary approach involves collaborating with various healthcare professionals such as podiatrists, endocrinologists, pain specialists, and physical therapists. This ensures a comprehensive assessment and comprehensive care plan for the patient.

2.2.9 Differential Diagnosis [8, 23]

Additional illnesses that can imitate DPN should be taken into account by the healthcare professional, such as nerve entrapment syndromes, autoimmune neuropathies, or drug-induced neuropathies. Ruling out these conditions is critical for accurate diagnosis.

Differential diagnosis is the process of distinguishing a particular disease or condition from other similar conditions based on a thorough evaluation of clinical features, symptoms, and diagnostic tests. DPN is a frequent diabetic complication, but it's important to think about additional potential reasons when assessing patients with neuropathic symptoms.

1. **Peripheral Neuropathies of Other Causes:**
   - Alcohol-related neuropathy: Peripheral neuropathy can be the result of chronic alcoholism, often presenting with a symmetric, length-dependent pattern similar to DPN.
   - Nutritional deficiencies: Deficiencies in vitamins, particularly B vitamins (B1, B6, B12), can cause peripheral neuropathy. Folate deficiency can also contribute.
   - Toxic neuropathies: Exposure to certain toxins, such as heavy metals or industrial chemicals, can result in neuropathy.
2. **Autoimmune Neuropathies:**
   - Guillain-Barré Syndrome (GBS): An acute, immune-mediated neuropathy that often follows an infection. It can lead to ascending weakness and sensory deficits.
   - Chronic inflammatory demyelinating polyneuropathy (CIDP): An autoimmune disorder characterized by chronic progressive or relapsing-remitting neuropathy.
3. **Infections:**
   - HIV-related neuropathy: Human immunodeficiency virus (HIV) can cause peripheral neuropathy, often presenting with a symmetric distal polyneuropathy.
   - Lyme disease: Lyme disease, caused by Borrelia burgdorferi, can lead to peripheral neuropathy if left untreated.
4. **Hereditary Neuropathies:**
   - Charcot-Marie-Tooth disease (CMT): A group of inherited neuropathies affecting the peripheral nerves, leading to muscle weakness and sensory loss.
   - Friedreich's ataxia: A genetic disorder that can result in peripheral neuropathy in addition to ataxia.
5. **Vasculitic Neuropathies:**
   - Polyarteritis nodosa (PAN): A systemic vasculitis affecting medium-sized arteries, which can lead to peripheral neuropathy.
   - Systemic lupus erythematosus (SLE): Lupus can involve the peripheral nervous system and cause neuropathy.
6. **Compression Neuropathies:**
   - Carpal tunnel syndrome: Compression of the median nerve at the wrist, leading to symptoms such as numbness and tingling in the hands.

- Peripheral nerve entrapments: Compression or entrapment of peripheral nerves at various locations, causing localized symptoms.

7. **Metabolic and Endocrine Causes:**
   - Hypothyroidism: Underactive thyroid function can lead to neuropathy.
   - Renal failure: Uremic neuropathy can be brought on by chronic renal disease.
8. **Medication-Induced Neuropathies:**
   - Certain medications, such as chemotherapy drugs, antiretrovirals, and certain antibiotics, can cause peripheral neuropathy as a side effect.

A thorough diagnosis frequently requires a mix of laboratory testing, physical examination, and clinical history, and sometimes nerve conduction studies or imaging studies. Collaborative efforts between neurologists, endocrinologists, and other specialists may be necessary for a comprehensive evaluation. The goal is to identify the underlying cause and tailor treatment accordingly.

2.2.10 Follow-Up

Regular follow-up assessments are essential because DPN is a progressive condition. Monitoring helps track changes in symptoms and allows for adjustments to the management plan as needed.

In conclusion, the assessment and diagnosis of DPN require a meticulous and multifaceted approach. Early detection, thorough evaluation, and ongoing monitoring are essential to manage this condition effectively and prevent complications. For DPN sufferers, a cooperative, interdisciplinary approach to treatment might be very beneficial, ensuring a more accurate diagnosis and a more comprehensive management plan.

2.3 Conclusion

In summary, this chapter on DPN assessment and diagnosis emphasizes the intricate nature of this prevalent complication in diabetes. The comprehensive evaluation integrates clinical, electrophysiological, and imaging methods to enhance diagnostic precision and guide effective management.

Clinical assessment, including a detailed medical history and neurological examinations, remains crucial for identifying DPN. Standardized screening tools and questionnaires aid in quantifying symptom severity. Electrophysiological studies, such as NCS and EMG, provide essential insights into objectively measuring nerve damage, while advanced imaging techniques offer non-invasive glimpses into structural changes in peripheral nerves.

Innovative methods like QST and skin biopsy address small fiber neuropathy nuances. Challenges persist, prompting ongoing research to refine diagnostics and explore novel biomarkers. The incorporation of artificial intelligence has the potential to improve diagnostic precision. In essence, a holistic approach that amalgamates clinical acumen with state-of-the-art diagnostic tools is imperative for early detection and targeted management of DPN. In addition to improving diagnosis accuracy, this multimodal approach paves the way for better patient outcomes and a greater standard of living for those coping with the hardships of DPN.

References

1. Petropoulos IN, Ponirakis G, Khan A, Almuhannadi H, Gad H, Malik RA. Diagnosing diabetic neuropathy: something old, something new. Diabetes Metab J. 2018;42(4):255–69.
2. Khramilin VN, Strokov IA, Davydov OS, Churyukanov MV. Diagnosis of diabetic polyneuropathy in primary care. Russ J Pain. 2021;19(2):47–59.
3. Boovaragasamy C, Gnanasabai G, Kumar M. A review on tools for measuring activity limitation in diabetic peripheral neuropathy. Int J Res Med Sci. 2021;10(1):285.
4. Snow K. Evaluation of Diabetic Peripheral Neuropathy (DPN): an overview. NEUROMetrix. 2012;1:1–12.
5. Wang X, Luo L, Xing J, Wang J, Shi B, Li YM, et al. Assessment of peripheral neuropathy in type 2 diabetes by diffusion tensor imaging. Quant Imaging Med Surg. 2022;12(1):395–405.
6. Oster JA. Diabetic peripheral neuropathy—patient examination guidelines for practitioners (part 2) [internet]. Myfootshop; 2019. p. 1–10. Available from: https://www.myfootshop.com/diabetic-peripheral-neuropathy-patient-examination-guidelines-for-practitioners.
7. Yang Z, Zhang Y, Chen R, Huang Y, Ji L, Sun F, et al. Simple tests to screen for diabetic peripheral neuropathy. Cochrane Database Syst Rev. 2018;2018(7):2–5.
8. Yu Y. Gold standard for diagnosis of DPN. Front Endocrinol (Lausanne). 2021;12(October):1–6.
9. Alahmar A. Quantitative sensory testing in type 1 diabetic patients with mild to severe diabetic neuropathy. J Res Med Dent Sci. 2016;4(2):105.
10. Sharma KNS, Kumar HA. Assessment of the diagnostic accuracy of Vibrasense compared to a biothesiometer and nerve conduction study for screening diabetic peripheral neuropathy. J Foot Ankle Res [Internet]. 2023;16(1):1–9. https://doi.org/10.1186/s13047-023-00667-3.
11. Bishop K, Poole R. Common tests for diabetic peripheral neuropathy. Pract Diabetes. 2022;39(6):35–8.
12. Gylfadottir SS, Weeracharoenkul D, Andersen ST, Niruthisard S, Suwanwalaikorn S, Jensen TS. Painful and non-painful diabetic polyneuropathy: clinical characteristics and diagnostic issues. J Diabetes Investig. 2019;10(5):1148–57.
13. Sharma S, Vas PR, Rayman G. Assessment of diabetic neuropathy using a point-of-care nerve conduction device shows significant associations with the ldiflare method and clinical neuropathy scoring. J Diabetes Sci Technol. 2015;9(1):123–31.
14. Dillingham T, Buschbacher R, Howard I, Malhotra G, Adkins SA, Lutteke W. AANEM reference values. AANEM practice topic; 2016. p. 371–7.
15. Kim JY, Kim E, Shim HS, Lee JH, Lee GJ, Kim K, et al. Reference standards for nerve conduction studies of individual nerves of lower extremity with expanded uncertainty in healthy Korean adults. Ann Rehabil Med. 2022;46(1):9–23.
16. Preston DC, Shapiro BE. Electromyography and neuromuscular disorders. 4th ed. Philadelphia, PA: Elsevier; 2021. 133, 247, 255 p

17. Rodriguez-Carreno I, Gila-Useros L, Malanda-Trigueros A. Motor unit action potential duration: measurement and significance [internet]. In: Advances in clinical neurophysiology; 2012. p. 1–27. Available from: https://www.intechopen.com/chapters/40104.
18. Zhou P, Rymer WZ. MUAP number estimates in surface EMG: template-matching methods and their performance boundaries. Ann Biomed Eng [Internet]. 2004;32(7):1007–15. https://doi.org/10.1023/B:ABME.0000032463.26331.b3.
19. Won JC, Park TS. Recent advances in diagnostic strategies for diabetic peripheral neuropathy. Endocrinol Metab. 2016;31(2):230–8.
20. Jiang X, Deng F, Rui S, Ma Y, Wang M, Deng B, et al. The evaluation of gait and balance for patients with early diabetic peripheral neuropathy: a cross-sectional study. Risk Manag Healthc Policy. 2022;15(March):543–52.
21. Bastyr EJ, Price KL, Bril V. Development and validity testing of the neuropathy total symptom score-6: questionnaire for the study of sensory symptoms of diabetic peripheral neuropathy. Clin Ther. 2005;27(8):1278–94.
22. Yang Z, Chen R, Zhang Y, Huang Y, Hong T, Sun F, et al. Scoring systems to screen for diabetic peripheral neuropathy. Cochrane Database Syst Rev. 2018;2018(7):1–21.
23. Sohn EH. Differential diagnosis of diabetic neuropathy. J Korean Diabetes [Internet]. 2010;11(3):183–7. https://doi.org/10.4093/kcd.2010.11.3.183.

Chapter 3
Quality of Life Questionnaires and Screening Scales for Diabetic Peripheral Neuropathy

Hina Vaish

Contents

3.1 Introduction

Neuropathy is the most prevalent complications of diabetes [1]. Diabetic peripheral neuropathy (DPN), characterized by persistent sensory signs and symptoms, is the most prevalent form [2].

Approximately, 50%–66% of people with diabetes mellitus will ultimately suffer from peripheral neuropathy in their lifetime [3].

H. Vaish (✉)
Department of Physiotherapy, School of Health Sciences, Chhatrapati Shahu Ji Maharaj University, Kanpur, Uttar Pradesh, India

© The Author(s), under exclusive license to Springer Nature Singapore Pte Ltd. 2024

M. Goyal, K. Goyal (eds.), *Rehabilitation in Diabetic Peripheral Neuropathy*,
https://doi.org/10.1007/978-981-97-9290-0_3

As the disease progresses, the symptoms may worsen, leaving patients vulnerable to complications such as diabetic ulceration and amputation. It is challenging to identify DPN during initial phases of the disease but it becomes extremely devastating once the substantial damage has occurred.

Peripheral neuropathy is commonly reported complications related to hyperglycemic conditions such as diabetes mellitus. As DPN commonly has devastating effects [4], early disease recognition will enable management and prevent long-standing adverse effects [5, 6]. Early identification of the disease is essential to avert complications and prevent influence on quality of life (QoL) [6, 7].

QoL is a significant concern linked to DPN treatment, and rapid assessment appears to be practical for use in clinical settings. Precise evaluation of QoL can be of benefit to both, the healthcare workforces and patients.

Numerous screening tools and QoL assessment methods are available for successful screening and disease assessment in adults with DPN.

To lessen the predicted impact that the diabetes will have in the coming years, early screening and intervention is essential. Diabetes has major effects on the body that are irreversible, thus, early recognition of associated adverse effects and its management is the key to achieve the best health outcomes.

This chapter further discusses the quality of life questionnaires and screening scales for DPN, their psychometric properties, available versions, and their scoring methods.

3.2 Quality of Life Questionnaires and Screening Scales

The tools to assess QoL in diabetic neuropathy population are presented in Fig. 3.1. Generic measures have been used such as SF 36, SF 12, and Nottingham Health Profile however, population specific questionnaires and scales are more accurate for evaluation of QoL in disease specific population.

3.2.1 Norfolk Quality of Life Diabetic Neuropathy Tool (QOL-DN)

QOL-DN is a validated tool to screen neuropathy. The tool was developed to discriminate between characteristic features present in DPN, such as variations in sensation in small and large fibers, besides characteristic changes to autonomic nervous system function [8, 9].

Norfolk QOL-DN identifies neuropathy in different populations like German and Romanian [10, 11]. QoL has been assessed using QOL-DN in clinical trials [12, 13]. Norfolk QOL-DN has been used to investigate the effect of neuropathy on QoL [10, 14–16].

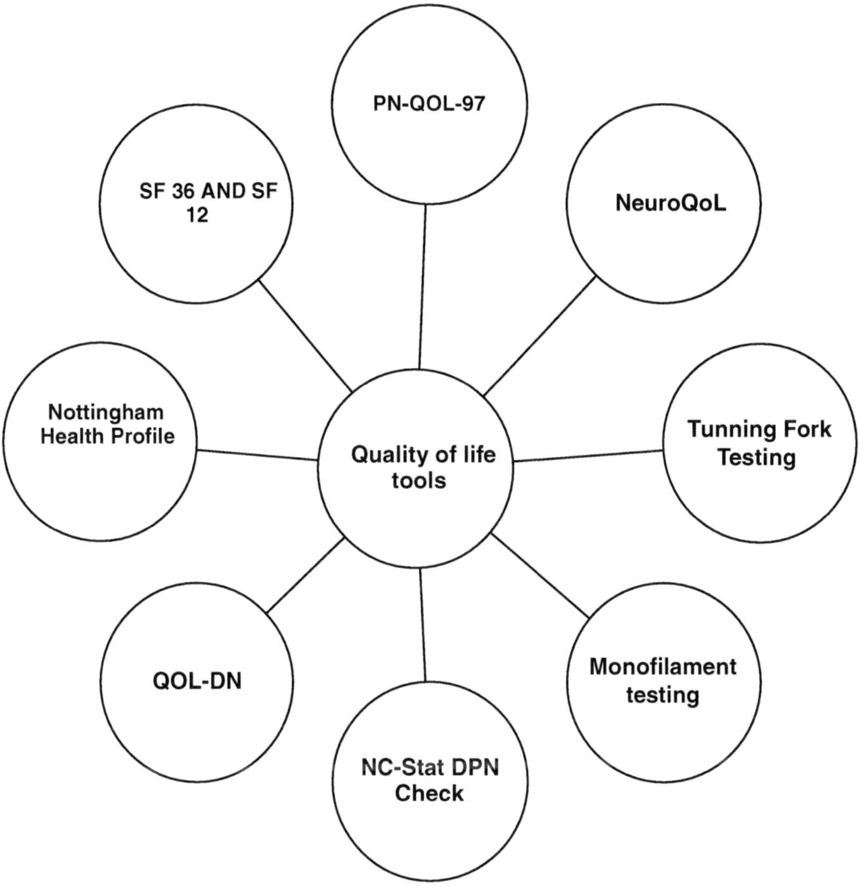

Fig. 3.1 Diabetic Peripheral Neuropathy Quality of life tools

3.2.1.1 Items

The questionnaire consists of 47 items.

The QOL-DN instrument has a total QOL score and five subscale Fig. 3.2.

3.2.1.2 Psychometric Properties

Total QoL scores were in correlation to total neuropathy scores. Intra-class correlation coefficients (ICC) were 0.9 for many domains. Cronbach's α for fiber specific domains were from 0.6 to 0.8 [9].

The criterion validity of the instrument has not been assessed.

The Norfolk QOL-DN was translated in German language. Overall QoL scores were different amongst individual five neuropathy groups [analysis of variance $p < 0.001$] [17].

3.2.1.3 Scoring

Total scores are calculated based on the scores for five domains evaluating symptoms and impacts of neuropathic health. Higher the scores, worse is the HRQoL [18] (Fig. 3.2).

3.2.2 *Peripheral Neuropathy Quality of Life Instrument (PN-QOL-97)*

Vickrey et al. developed PN-QOL-97 to assess peripheral neuropathy [19]. Initial tool had 162 items. The tool was re-evaluated, and the items were reduced from 162 to 97 (Fig. 3.3).

3.2.2.1 Items

The scale includes 97 items. A total of 91 items are presented among 16 scales with multiple items [19].

3.2.2.2 Psychometric Properties

PN-QOL-97 is a validated tool for use in diabetic neuropathy (DN) population. Test-retest reliability had been established [19].

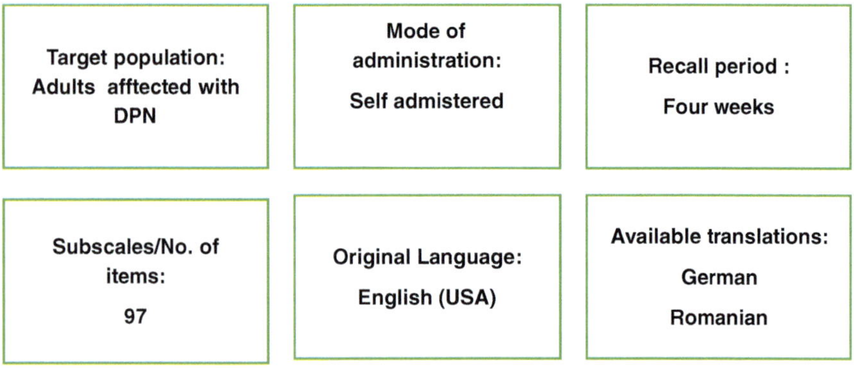

Fig. 3.2 Characteristic of the Norfolk Quality of Life Diabetic Neuropathy Tool [9]

3.2.2.3 Scoring

The physical and mental components are scored by calculations provided by the author [19] (Fig. 3.3).

3.2.3 *Neuropathy-and Foot Ulcer-Specific Quality of Life Instrument (NeuroQoL)*

The NeuroQoL was designed to measure QoL and is neuropathy-and foot ulcer-specific instrument [20].

3.2.3.1 Items

The NeuroQoL has 28 items with three physical domains, two psychosocial domains and one overall measure of QoL. Reliability (test-retest) and validity (criterion) were not presented in the main study (Fig. 3.4).

3.2.3.2 Psychometric Properties

Reliability of the scales ranges from 0.86 to 0.95. Floor effects were reported to be modest. Less evidence of ceiling effects was reported. NeuroQoL physical scale and psychosocial scale had moderate correlation ($r = 0.39–0.67$) [20].

The research demonstrated link between neuropathy symptoms and depressive symptoms using NeuroQoL [21].

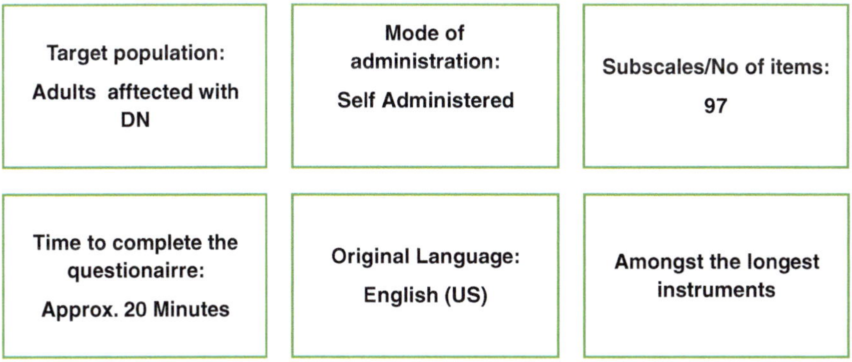

Fig. 3.3 Characteristics of Peripheral Neuropathy Quality of Life Instrument (PN-QOL-97) [19]

NeuroQoL is reliable and valid tool for diabetic population to assess neuropathy symptoms [22]. Researches revealed validity of NeuroQoL by detection of variations in the DN severity [23].

The NeuroQoL has widely been used in DN related research [24].

NeuroQoL has been translated into Hindi language (NeuroQoL-H). Overall score of validated NeuroQoL-H in diabetes mellitus population is 60. For all the items in Hindi version of NeuroQoL, item-level content validity index (I-CVI) ≥ 0.8 and scale level content validity index (S-CVI) = 0.95. The floor effect is reported to be 24% and the reported ceiling effect was 1% [25].

NeuroQoL has been translated and validated into Brazilian Portuguese as a reliable instrument [26].

3.2.3.3 Scoring

The questions from 1 to 27 have response options of two categories: frequency of symptoms in past 4 weeks and how much bother did this cause you? [20].

Question A–F have response options of very much, quite a lot, somewhat, a little, not at all [20].

Question 28 is related to overall effect of foot problem on quality of life with response options ranging from very much to not at all. Question 29 is about overall QoL with options ranging from excellent to poor [20] (Fig. 3.4, Table 3.1).

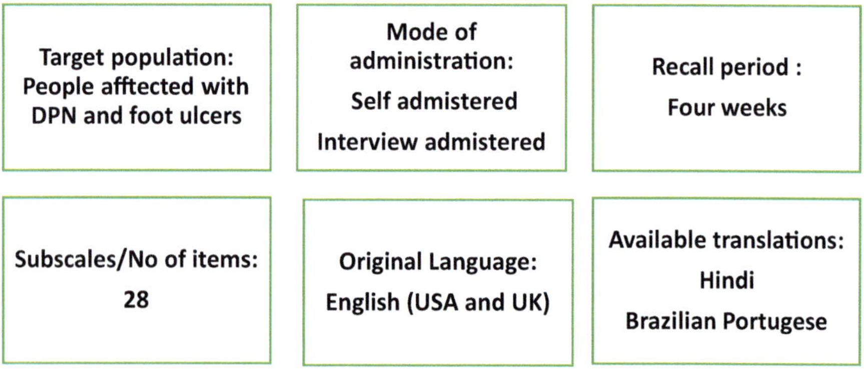

Fig. 3.4 Characteristics of neuropathy and foot ulcer-specific quality of life instrument (NeuroQoL) [20]

Table 3.1 Psychometric properties of quality of life questionnaires and screening scales

Scale	Internal consistency	Test–retest reliability
QOL-DN [9]	Cronbach's α 0.60–0.80 for all three groups (DPN population, diabetic controls and for healthy controls)	ICC > 0.8 for all scales andOverall score (4–6 weeks)ICC > 0.9 (1–3-month intervals)
PN-QOL-97 [19]	Cronbach's α 0.67–0.93 (median 0.88); all >0.70 except for sleep scale (0.67)	ICCs: 0.42–0.84 (median 0.77); all >0.67 except stigma
NeuroQoL [20]	Cronbach's α: 5 scales 0.86–0.95	Not reported in main study.

3.3 Health–Related Quality of Life in Patients with Diabetic Foot Ulcers

Diabetic foot ulcer (DFU) is commonly seen in diabetes patients, with adverse effects on patients' HRQol. There are tools available for assessment of QoL in DFU population (Table 3.2).

3.3.1 The Diabetic Foot Ulcer Scale (DFS)

DFS was designed for population with diabetic foot ulcers (DFUs) [27].

3.3.1.1 Items

DFS consist of 54 items, 15 quality of life subscales.

3.3.1.2 Psychometric Properties

The DFS has good internal consistency along with adequate reliability (test-retest) [27]. All scales exhibited item discriminant validity of ≥85%. Over 85% of the items satisfied the required level of homogeneity.

3.3.1.3 Scoring

The participants mark responses on a 5-point scale. A higher QoL among diabetic foot ulcers individuals is indicated a higher score.

Table 3.2 Comparison of DFS and DFS-SF

Criteria	DFS	DFS-SF
Subscales	15 [27]	06 [28]
Original language	English [27]	English [28]
Available translations	—	Chinese [29], Mandarin Chinese [30], Spanish [31], Korean [32], Turkish [33], Greek [34], Polish [35], Persian [36], Brazilian [37], Malayalam [38].

3.3.2 Diabetic Foot Ulcer Scale–Short Form (DFS–SF)

DFS-SF was made for patients with DFUs [28].

3.3.2.1 Items

DFS–SF has 29 items and there are 6 subscales [28].

3.3.2.2 Psychometric Properties

Chinese DFS-SF's Cronbach's α is 0.8–0.92. It has item-scale correlation of 0.63–0.84. It has good construct validity [29].

The DFU-SF Mandarin Chinese version has Cronbach's α value of 0.952, I-CVI of 0.800–1.000, and average S-CVI (S-CVI/Ave) of 0.911. The criterion-related validity has also been tested ($p < 0.05$) [30].

The Spanish version of DFU-SF has Cronbach's α of 0.720–0.948. Excellent reproducibility has been demonstrated by the DFS-SF domains (ICC ranged from 0.77 to 0.92). The criterion validity of Spanish version of DFS-SF is good ($p < 0.001$) [31].

Cronbach's α > 0.70 for all scales of Korean version of DFU-SF. Spearman's correlations show construct validity [32].

The Turkish version of the DFS-SF is validated measure to access QOL of diabetic foot population. The Content Validity Index (CVI) is 0.97, factor loading of scale is reported to be 0.378–0.982, and Cronbach's α of 0.81–0.94 [33].

The Greek version of DFS-SF is suitable for evaluating QoL in patients with DFU with Cronbach's α > 0.70 for all scales. The item convergence rate is excellent (100%) and good discrimination rates (84.1%) [34].

The Polish DFS-SF scales has Cronbach's α of 0.82–0.93), good construct validity and satisfactory item convergent and discriminant validity [35].

The Persian version DFS-SF has adequate internal consistency shown by Cronbach's α = 0.89 and ICC > 0.69 and the composite reliability ≥0.70 for all dimensions [36].

The Brazilian DFS-SF version has Cronbach's α > 0.70 and good convergent validity [31, 37].

The Cronbach's-α of the Malayalam version of the DFS-SF questionnaire varied from 0.990 to 0.996, indicating high reliability. The average CVI score was 1.00. Dependency and VAS have a positive association ($r = 0.538$), while ulcer care and VAS have a negative correlation ($r = 0.494$) [38].

3.3.2.3 Scoring

The participants mark responses on a Likert scale (5 point). A higher QoL among diabetic foot ulcers individuals is indicated a higher score [28].

3.3.3 Cardiff Wound Impact Scale (CWIS)

The Cardiff Wound Impact Scale (CWIS) is used in population of chronic wounds and ulcers with the goal of achieving both DFU and wound-related HRQoL [39].

3.3.3.1 Item

CWIS has three subscales: [39].

- Physical symptoms and everyday living containing 12 items
- Social life contains seven items
- Well-being contains seven items

3.3.3.2 Psychometric Properties

Each of the subscales have Cronbach's α > 0·75 indicating high internal consistency of CWIS [39].

Apart from its construct validity, the Spanish translation of the CWIS demonstrates adequate psychometric properties [40].

CWIS is available in Brazilian-Portuguese. It has satisfactory face validity and content validity [41].

The linguistic validation of CWIS is available for Chinses, Dutch, French, German, US English, and Swedish population; also validated for Canadian population [42–45].

3.3.3.3 Scoring

For each scale, the items are added together to get the scale scores. Each of the three scales is then converted into a scale from 0 to 100. A greater score is indicative of a positive rating [39].

3.4 Scale to Detect Diabetic Neuropathic Pain

Neuropathic pain occurs commonly is diabetic neuropathy [4, 46]. There are several scales available for detection of diabetic neuropathic pain as listed in Fig. 3.1 (Fig. 3.5) (Table 3.3).

3.4.1 Leeds Assessment of Neuropathic Symptoms and Signs (LANSS)

LANSS was developed in 2001 by Bennett [47].

3.4.1.1 Items

It comprises of seven item pain scale: five symptom related questions and two examination items.

3.4.1.2 Psychometric Properties

LANSS is a validated and reliable scale. LANSS has sensitivity of 85% and specificity of is reported to be 80%. LANSS demonstrates Cronbach's α of 0.74 [47].

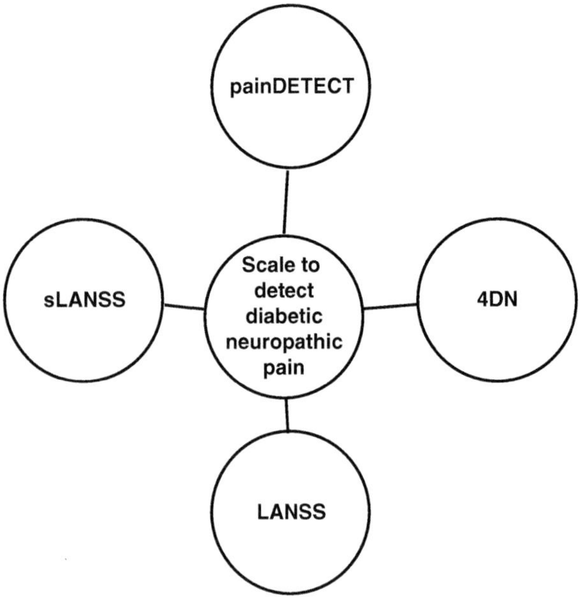

Fig. 3.5 Scale to detect diabetic neuropathic pain

Table 3.3 Characteristics of scale to detect diabetic neuropathic pain

Name of tool	Language of original version	Available version
LANSS	English [47]	Turkish [48], Portugese [49]
s-LANSS	English [50]	
	Arabic [51], Turkish [52]	
DN 4	French [53]	Turkish [54], Arabic [55] Nepalese [56], Spanish [57]
painDETECT	English [56]	Turkish [60], Arabic [63] , Korean [62], Persian [61], and Japanese [59]

LANSS has been translated into Turkish as a validity and reliable tool. It has sensitivity of 89.9% and specificity of 94.2%. LANSS gave an accurate diagnosis ratio and the kappa value of 0.841 [48].

The Portuguese translation of LANSS is available as a reliable tool with Cronbach's $\alpha = 0.78$. Its sensitivity and specificity are 89% and 74%, respectively [49].

3.4.1.3 Scoring

The score ranges from 0 to 24. A score ≥ 12 indicates pain of predominantly neuropathic origin.

3.4.2 self-Leeds Assessment of Neuropathic Symptoms and Signs (sLANSS)

sLANSS was developed by Bennet by revising the examination portions of LANSS so that patients can apply these steps to themselves [50].

3.4.2.1 Items

It comprises of seven questions. It contains five questions regarding sensory symptoms and two sensory self-examination items related to allodynia and altered pinprick threshold [50].

3.4.2.2 Psychometric Properties

- sLANSS has accuracy of 80%, 74% of sensitivity, and 76% of specificity [50].
- sLANSS has been translated, culturally adapted, and validated in Arabic. Cronbach's α for Arabic sLANSS was 0.72. Arabic sLANSS has good measure-

ment of agreement of individual items with kappa coefficients ranged 0.462–1.00 [51].

The questionnaire has been translated in Turkish with correlation coefficient of 0.97 ($P < 0.01$). It has sensitivity of 72.3% and specificity of 80.4% [52].

3.4.2.3 Scoring

The scores are in the range of 0–24. A score of 12 or higher indicates mostly neuropathic pain.

3.4.3 *Douleur Neuropathique 4 (4DN)*

Bouhassira developed DN4 in French in 2005 [53]. The instrument was validated in Turkish language in 2010 [54].

3.4.3.1 Items

4DN has ten items under four titles including examination of llodynia and hyperalgesia. The questionnaire's first seven questions assess sensory characteristics and the rest of the three items are for clinical examination [53].

3.4.3.2 Psychometric Properties

The Arabic translation and validation of DN4 has been done. It has a diagnostic accuracy; specificity of 74.5% and sensitivity of 88.3% [55].

The DN4 has been translated and is a valid tool for the Nepalese with 75% sensitivity and 95.3% specificity. The internal consistency was 0.710 with good test–retest reliability was (ICC = 0.877) [56].

The DN4 has been translated and validated into Spanish language. It is a reliable [Cronbach's α coefficient: 0.71, ICC: 0.80 (0.71–0.89), and test–retest ICC: 0.95 (0.92–0.97)] and valid instrument [57].

The Turkish translation of DN4 is a reliable questionnaire for neuropathic pain population, with Cronbach's α of 0.97 (ranged from 0.93 to 1.00). It has good test and retest reliability, with a high ICC of 0.95 [54].

3.4.3.3 Scoring

Total score is out of 10. A neuropathic origin is suggested by a score of 4 or higher.

3.4.4 painDETECT

painDETECT scale was developed in 2006; it includes questions related to symptoms, type, severity, and radiation of pain [58].

3.4.4.1 Items

It comprises of three items with total of nine questions: Seven questions of gradation of pain, one question each of pain course pattern, and radiation of pain, respectively.

3.4.4.2 Psychometric Properties

The painDETECT is a reliable instrument and has a high sensitivity and specificity [58].

Turkish validation was done in 2013, Cronbach's $\alpha = 0.81$ [59]. Turkish painDETECT is correlated with LANSS (r=0.89) and DN4 (r=0.82) [60].

The scale has also been translated into Japanese (Cronbach α for the total score was 0.78 and ICC = 0.94), Persian (Cronbach's α and ICC were 0.76 and 0.97, respectively), Korean (Cronbach's α of 0.84), and Arabic (ICC of 0.970, Cronbach's α values 0.684) [59, 61–63].

3.4.4.3 Scoring

For each question of gradation of pain, the score ranges from 0 to 5.

For pain course pattern the score range includes −1, 0, and + 1.

For pain radiation the scores are +2 / 0.

The total score ranged from 0 to 38.

Score < 12 represents nociceptive pain.

Score of 13–18 represents possible neuropathic pain.

Score ≥ 19 represents >90% likelihood of neuropathic pain (Table 3.3).

3.5 Summary

All the instruments for assessing QoL in DPN in diabetic foot ulcers and detecting diabetic neuropathic pain provides evidence for their use in clinical settings. All scales and questionnaires are supported by evidence of reliability and validity though test–retest reliability lacks in few and data on responsiveness is limited. The choice of instrument to be used should primarily focus on the purpose of use and may depend on the setting and language of use.

References

1. Galiero R, Caturano A, Vetrano E, et al. Peripheral neuropathy in diabetes mellitus: pathogenetic mechanisms and diagnostic options. Int J Mol Sci. 2023;24(4):3554. https://doi.org/10.3390/ijms24043554.
2. Smith SC, Lamping DL, Maclaine GD. Measuring health-related quality of life in diabetic peripheral neuropathy: a systematic review. Diabetes Res Clin Pract. 2012;96(3):261–70. https://doi.org/10.1016/j.diabres.2011.11.013.
3. Bodman MA, Varacallo M. Peripheral diabetic neuropathy. In: StatPearls [Internet]. Treasure Island (FL): StatPearls Publishing; 2023. Available from: https://www.ncbi.nlm.nih.gov/books/NBK442009/.
4. Vinik AI, Nevoret ML, Casellini C, Parson H. Diabetic neuropathy. Endocrinol Metab Clin N Am. 2013;42(4):747–87. https://doi.org/10.1016/j.ecl.2013.06.001.
5. Eikenberg JD, Davy BM. Prediabetes: a prevalent and treatable, but often unrecognized, clinical condition. J Acad Nutr Diet. 2013;113(2):213–8. https://doi.org/10.1016/j.jand.2012.10.018.
6. Papanas N, Ziegler D. Prediabetic neuropathy: does it exist? Curr Diab Rep. 2012;12(4):376–83. https://doi.org/10.1007/s11892-012-0278-3.
7. Ferrannini E, Gastaldelli A, Iozzo P. Pathophysiology of prediabetes. Med Clin North Am. 2011;95(2):327–39. https://doi.org/10.1016/j.mcna.2010.11.005.
8. Vinik EJ, Hayes C, Oglesby A, Vinik AI. Identification of factors in the nerve fiber specific quality of life (QOL-DN) inventory that reflect QOL and health status. Diabetes. 2004;53:A295.
9. Vinik EJ, Hayes RP, Oglesby A, et al. The development and validation of the Norfolk QOL-DN, a new measure of patients' perception of the effects of diabetes and diabetic neuropathy. Diabetes Technol Ther. 2005;7(3):497–508. https://doi.org/10.1089/dia.2005.7.497.
10. Vinik AI, Shapiro DY, Rauschkolb C, et al. A randomized withdrawal, placebo-controlled study evaluating the efficacy and tolerability of tapentadol extended release in patients with chronic painful diabetic peripheral neuropathy. Diabetes Care. 2014;37(8):2302–9. https://doi.org/10.2337/dc13-2291.
11. Veresiu AI, Bondor CI, Florea B, et al. Detection of undisclosed neuropathy and assessment of its impact on quality of life: a survey in 25,000 Romanian patients with diabetes. J Diabetes Complicat. 2015;29(5):644–9. https://doi.org/10.1016/j.jdiacomp.2015.04.001.
12. Boyd A, Casselini C, Vinik E, Vinik A. Quality of life and objective measures of diabetic neuropathy in a prospective placebo-controlled trial of ruboxistaurin and topiramate. J Diabetes Sci Technol. 2011;5(3):714–22.
13. Casellini CM, Barlow PM, Rice AL, et al. A 6-month, randomized, double-masked, placebo-controlled study evaluating the effects of the protein kinase C-beta inhibitor ruboxistaurin on skin microvascular blood flow and other measures of diabetic peripheral neuropathy. Diabetes Care. 2007;30(4):896–902. https://doi.org/10.2337/dc06-1699.
14. Coelho T, Maia LF, da Silva AM, et al. Long-term effects of tafamidis for the treatment of transthyretin familial amyloid polyneuropathy. J Neurol. 2013;260(11):2802–14. https://doi.org/10.1007/s00415-013-7051-7.
15. Coelho T, Maia LF, Martins da Silva A, et al. Tafamidis for transthyretin familial amyloid polyneuropathy: a randomized, controlled trial. Neurology. 2012;79(8):785–92. https://doi.org/10.1212/WNL.0b013e3182661eb1.
16. Vinik E, Silva M, Vinik A. Relationship between quality of life and health-related measures including symptoms, biochemical markers and tumor burden. Pancreas. 2010;39(2):282.
17. Vinik EJ, Paulson JF, Ford-Molvik SL, Vinik AI. German-translated Norfolk quality of life (QOL-DN) identifies the same factors as the English version of the tool and discriminates different levels of neuropathy severity. J Diabetes Sci Technol. 2008;2(6):1075–86. https://doi.org/10.1177/193229680800200616.
18. Yarlas A, Lovley A, Brown D, Kosinski M, Vera-Llonch M. Responder analysis for neuropathic impairment and quality-of-life assessment in patients with hereditary transthyretin

amyloidosis with polyneuropathy in the NEURO-TTR study. J Neurol. 2022;269(1):323–35. https://doi.org/10.1007/s00415-021-10635-1.
19. Vickrey BG, Hays RD, Beckstrand M. Development of a health-related quality of life measure for peripheral neuropathy. Neurorehabil Neural Repair. 2000;14(2):93–104. https://doi.org/10.1177/154596830001400202.
20. Vileikyte L, Peyrot M, Bundy C, Rubin RR, Leventhal H, Mora P, Shaw JE, Baker P, Boulton AJ. The development and validation of a neuropathy-and foot ulcer-specific quality of life instrument. Diabetes Care. 2003;26(9):2549–55.
21. Vileikyte L, Leventhal H, Gonzalez JS, et al. Diabetic peripheral neuropathy and depressive symptoms: the association revisited. Diabetes Care. 2005;28(10):2378–83. https://doi.org/10.2337/diacare.28.10.2378.
22. Bergis N, Hermanns N, Kulzer B. Erfassung von symptomatik und lebensqualität bei diabetischer neuropathie. [The assessment of symptomatology and quality of life in diabetic neuropathy]. Verhaltenstherapie & Verhaltensmedizin. 2011;32(4):365–75.
23. Vileikyte L, Peyrot M, Gonzalez JS, Rubin R, Ulbrecht J, Leventhal H, Cavanagh P, Boulton A. Longitudinal validation of the neuropathy and foot ulcer-specific-quality of life instrument (NeuroQoL). Diabetes. 2007;56:A80.
24. Lavery LA, Murdoch DP, Williams J, Lavery DC. Does anodyne light therapy improve peripheral neuropathy in diabetes? A double-blind, sham-controlled, randomized trial to evaluate monochromatic infrared photoenergy. Diabetes Care. 2008;31(2):316–21. https://doi.org/10.2337/dc07-1794.
25. Saraf A, Goyal M, Vileikyte L, Ateef M, Samuel AJ. Neuropathy-and foot-ulcer specific quality of life instrument (NeuroQoL): translation, cross-cultural adaptation and content validation in Hindi. Foot Ankle Surg. 2023;29(2):105–10. https://doi.org/10.1016/j.fas.2022.11.003.
26. Xavier AT, Foss MC, Marques Junior W, dos Santos CB, Onofre PT, Pace AE. Cultural adaptation and validation of the neuropathy—and foot ulcer—specific quality of life instrument (NeuroQol) for Brazilian Portuguese—phase 1. Rev Lat Am Enfermagem. 2011;19(6):1352–61. https://doi.org/10.1590/s0104-11692011000600011.
27. Abetz L, Sutton M, Brady L, McNulty P, Gagnon DD. The diabetic foot ulcer scale (DFS): a quality of life instrument for use in clinical trials. Pract Diabetes Int. 2002;19(6):167–75.
28. Bann CM, Fehnel SE, Gagnon DD. Development and validation of the diabetic foot ulcer scale-short form (DFS-SF). PharmacoEconomics. 2003;21(17):1277–90. https://doi.org/10.2165/00019053-200321170-00004.
29. Hui LF, Yee-Tak Fong D, Yam M, Yuk IW. Translation and validation of the Chinese diabetic foot ulcer scale—short form. Patient. 2008;1(2):137–45. https://doi.org/10.2165/01312067-200801020-00009.
30. Ma L, Ma W, Lin S, Li Y, Ran X. Adaptation and validation of the diabetic foot ulcer scale-short form scale for Chinese diabetic foot ulcers individuals. Int J Environ Res Public Health. 2022;19(21):14568. https://doi.org/10.3390/ijerph192114568.
31. Martinez-Gonzalez D, Dòria M, Martínez-Alonso M, et al. Adaptation and validation of the diabetic foot ulcer scale-short form in Spanish subjects [published correction appears in J Clin Med. 2022 Oct 10;11(19)]. J Clin Med. 2020;9(8):2497. https://doi.org/10.3390/jcm9082497.
32. Lee YN. Translation and validation of the Korean version of the diabetic foot ulcer scale-short form. Int Wound J. 2019;16 Suppl 1(Suppl 1):3–12. https://doi.org/10.1111/iwj.13025.
33. Toygar İ, Hançerlioğlu S, Gül S, Utku T, Şimşir IY, Çetinkalp Ş. Turkish adaptation of diabetic foot ulcer scale–short form. Int J Low Extrem Wounds. 2020;19(3):269–74. https://doi.org/10.1177/1534734620921036.
34. Kontodimopoulos N, Veniou A, Tentolouris N, Niakas D. Validity and reliability of the Greek version of the diabetic foot ulcer scale—short form (DFS-SF). Hormones (Athens). 2016;15(3):394–403. https://doi.org/10.14310/horm.2002.1682.
35. Macioch T, Sobol E, Krakowiecki A, Mrozikiewicz-Rakowska B, Kasprowicz M, Hermanowski T. Health related quality of life in patients with diabetic foot ulceration—translation and polish

adaptation of diabetic foot ulcer scale short form. Health Qual Life Outcomes. 2017;15(1):15. https://doi.org/10.1186/s12955-017-0587-y.
36. Tavassolmand SS, Montazeri A, Madadizadeh F, Dehghan HR, Ranjbar M, Ameri H. Translation and validation of the Persian version of diabetic foot ulcer scaleshort form (DFS-SF). Int Wound J. 2023;20(3):822–30. https://doi.org/10.1111/iwj.13929.
37. de Oliveira Kaizer UA, Alexandre NMC, Rodrigues RCM, Cornélio ME, de Melo Lima MH, São-João TM. Measurement properties and factor analysis of the diabetic foot ulcer scale-short form (DFS-SF). Int Wound J. 2020;17(3):670–82. https://doi.org/10.1111/iwj.13310.
38. Raju BN, Mateti UV, Mohan R, D'Souza C, Shastry CS, D'Souza N. Transcultural adaptation of the Malayalam version of the diabetic foot ulcer scale-short form. Clin Epidemiol Global Health. 2022;18:101190.
39. Price P, Harding K. Cardiff wound impact schedule: the development of a condition-specific questionnaire to assess health-related quality of life in patients with chronic wounds of the lower limb. Int Wound J. 2004;1(1):10–7. https://doi.org/10.1111/j.1742-481x.2004.00007.x.
40. Granado-Casas M, Martinez-Gonzalez D, Martínez-Alonso M, et al. Psychometric validation of the Cardiff wound impact schedule questionnaire in a Spanish population with diabetic foot ulcer. J Clin Med. 2021;10(17):4023. https://doi.org/10.3390/jcm10174023.
41. Augusto FDS, Blanes L, Nicodemo D, Ferreira LM. Translation and cross-cultural adaptation of the Cardiff wound impact schedule to Brazilian Portuguese. J Tissue Viability. 2017;26(2):113–8. https://doi.org/10.1016/j.jtv.2016.12.002.
42. Huang Y, Wu M, Xing P, et al. Translation and validation of the Chinese Cardiff wound impact schedule. Int J Low Extrem Wounds. 2014;13(1):5–11. https://doi.org/10.1177/1534734614521233.
43. Acquadro C, Price P, Wollina U. Linguistic validation of the Cardiff wound impact schedule into French, German and US English. J Wound Care. 2005;14(1):14–7. https://doi.org/10.12968/jowc.2005.14.1.26713.
44. Fagerdahl AM, Boström L, Ulfvarson J, Bergström G, Ottosson C. Translation and validation of the wound-specific quality of life instrument Cardiff wound impact schedule in a Swedish population. Scand J Caring Sci. 2014;28(2):398–404. https://doi.org/10.1111/scs.12050.
45. van Doorn LP, Sijberden JP, Brouwers JJWM, Goossens LD, Hamming JF. Validation of the Dutch translation of the Cardiff wound impact schedule for evaluation of the health-related quality of life of patients with chronic wounds. Int Wound J. 2020;17(5):1225–30. https://doi.org/10.1111/iwj.13388.
46. Colloca L, Ludman T, Bouhassira D, et al. Neuropathic pain. Nat Rev Dis Primers. 2017;3:17002. https://doi.org/10.1038/nrdp.2017.2.
47. Bennett M. The LANSS pain scale: the Leeds assessment of neuropathic symptoms and signs. Pain. 2001;92(1–2):147–57. https://doi.org/10.1016/s0304-3959(00)00482-6.
48. Yucel A, Senocak M, Kocasoy Orhan E, Cimen A, Ertas M. Results of the Leeds assessment of neuropathic symptoms and signs pain scale in Turkey: a validation study. J Pain. 2004;5(8):427–32. https://doi.org/10.1016/j.jpain.2004.07.001.
49. Barbosa M, Bennett MI, Verissimo R, Carvalho D. Cross-cultural psychometric assessment of the Leeds assessment of neuropathic symptoms and signs (LANSS) pain scale in the Portuguese population. Pain Pract. 2014;14(7):620–4. https://doi.org/10.1111/papr.12118.
50. Bennett MI, Smith BH, Torrance N, Potter J. The S-LANSS score for identifying pain of predominantly neuropathic origin: validation for use in clinical and postal research. J Pain. 2005;6(3):149–58. https://doi.org/10.1016/j.jpain.2004.11.007.
51. Elzahaf RA, Tashani OA, Unsworth BA, Johnson MI. Translation and linguistic validation of the self-completed Leeds assessment of neuropathic symptoms and signs (S-LANSS) scale for use in a Libyan population. Pain Pract. 2013;13(3):198–205. https://doi.org/10.1111/j.1533-2500.2012.00576.x.
52. Koc R, Erdemoglu AK. Validity and reliability of the Turkish self-administered Leeds assessment of neuropathic symptoms and signs (S-LANSS) questionnaire. Pain Med. 2010;11(7):1107–14. https://doi.org/10.1111/j.1526-4637.2010.00837.x.

53. Bouhassira D, Attal N, Alchaar H, et al. Comparison of pain syndromes associated with nervous or somatic lesions and development of a new neuropathic pain diagnostic questionnaire (DN4). Pain. 2005;114(1–2):29–36. https://doi.org/10.1016/j.pain.2004.12.010.
54. Unal-Cevik I, Sarioglu-Ay S, Evcik D. A comparison of the DN4 and LANSS questionnaires in the assessment of neuropathic pain: validity and reliability of the Turkish version of DN4. J Pain. 2010;11(11):1129–35. https://doi.org/10.1016/j.jpain.2010.02.003.
55. Terkawi AS, Abolkhair A, Didier B, et al. Development and validation of Arabic version of the douleur neuropathique 4 questionnaire. Saudi J Anaesth. 2017;11(Suppl 1):S31–9. https://doi.org/10.4103/sja.SJA_97_17.
56. Shakya BM, Shrestha A, Poudyal AK, et al. Nepalese version of Douleur Neuropathique 4 (DN4) questionnaire for detection of neuropathic pain signs and symptoms: translation and psychometric properties. PLoS One. 2023;18(7):e0287737. https://doi.org/10.1371/journal.pone.0287737.
57. Perez C, Galvez R, Huelbes S, et al. Validity and reliability of the Spanish version of the DN4 (Douleur Neuropathique 4 questions) questionnaire for differential diagnosis of pain syndromes associated to a neuropathic or somatic component. Health Qual Life Outcomes. 2007;5:66. https://doi.org/10.1186/1477-7525-5-66.
58. Freynhagen R, Baron R, Gockel U, Tölle TR. painDETECT: a new screening questionnaire to identify neuropathic components in patients with back pain. Curr Med Res Opin. 2006;22(10):1911–20. https://doi.org/10.1185/030079906X132488.
59. Matsubayashi Y, Takeshita K, Sumitani M, et al. Validity and reliability of the Japanese version of the painDETECT questionnaire: a multicenter observational study. PLoS One. 2013;8(9):e68013. https://doi.org/10.1371/journal.pone.0068013.
60. Alkan H, Ardic F, Erdogan C, Sahin F, Sarsan A, Findikoglu G. Turkish version of the painDETECT questionnaire in the assessment of neuropathic pain: a validity and reliability study. Pain Med. 2013;14(12):1933–43. https://doi.org/10.1111/pme.12222.
61. Ghamkhar L, Saghaeian SM, Niknam H, Hashemi SM, Freynhagen R, Kahlaee AH. Cross-cultural adaptation and validation of the Persian version of the painDETECT questionnaire. Curr Med Res Opin. 2021;37(12):2133–9. https://doi.org/10.1080/03007995.2021.1980778.
62. Sung JK, Choi JH, Jeong J, et al. Korean version of the painDETECT questionnaire: a study for cultural adaptation and validation. Pain Pract. 2017;17(4):494–504. https://doi.org/10.1111/papr.12472.
63. Abu-Shaheen A, Yousef S, Riaz M, et al. Testing the validity and reliability of the Arabic version of the painDETECT questionnaire in the assessment of neuropathic pain. PLoS One. 2018;13(4):e0194358. https://doi.org/10.1371/journal.pone.

Chapter 4
Non-pharmacological Treatment Interventions in Management of Diabetic Peripheral Neuropathy

Aakansha Saraf

Contents

4.1 Introduction

Diabetic neuropathy (DN) is a unique degenerative condition affecting the peripheral nervous system, specifically focusing on sensory and autonomic axons initially, followed by a lesser impact on motor axons [1]. DN is the most prevalent and intricate side effect of diabetes mellitus [2].

Peripheral neuropathic pain (PNP) refers to pain stemming from neuropathic origins, typically originating from a lesion or chronic condition impacting the peripheral nervous system [3]. When peripheral nerve dysfunction symptoms are present in a diabetic patient after all other potential causes have been ruled out, the condition is known as peripheral nerve dysfunction (DN), which is an exclusive consequence [1]. It is the typical reason for non-traumatic amputation and related

A. Saraf (✉)
Physiotherapist, Sahara Physiotherapy Clinic, Gold Coast, QLD, Australia

© The Author(s), under exclusive license to Springer Nature Singapore Pte Ltd. 2024

M. Goyal, K. Goyal (eds.), *Rehabilitation in Diabetic Peripheral Neuropathy*,
https://doi.org/10.1007/978-981-97-9290-0_4

hospitalization [4]. Diabetic autonomic neuropathy results in mortality and morbidity leading to silent myocardial infarction decreasing longevity. It is estimated that diabetes patients, almost two-third have clinical of subclinical neuropathy. Electrodiagnostic testing and nerve conduction studies helps in the diagnosis of neuropathy. The prevalence of neuropathy increases with the continuation of diabetes mellitus. The occurrence of neuropathy is common irrespective of the type of diabetes. DM and related complications reduce the standard of living of patients suffering of the disease [5]. Based on approximations, neuropathic pain prevalence in the general population ranges from 3% to 17% [6].

Therefore, in order to alleviate the suffering of patients, interventions should transition from merely suppressing symptoms to implementing a disease-modifying approach. DN has a remarkably high illness burden. Less than half of individuals experiencing neuropathic pain find relief through pharmacological interventions, leaving a considerable portion untreated or inadequately treated despite the availability of various pharmaceutical medications and management guidelines for chronic neuropathic pain. Therefore, it's the need of the hour for novel therapeutics that can be used either alone or in conjunction with existing treatments. It's crucial to advance the development of innovative, last-resort interventional therapeutic treatments to provide relief for patients who remain unresponsive to conventional interventions. Non-pharmacological treatment interventions have been highly neglected, but they have an effectual importance in the treatment of diabetes peripheral neuropathy [7]. The non-pharmacological intervention is spinal cord stimulation, magnetic stimulation, photon stimulation among others. This chapter will delve into a comprehensive examination of the mechanisms and effectiveness of non-pharmacological interventions in treating diabetic peripheral neuropathy (DPN).

4.2 Diabetic Neuropathic Pain

Diabetic neuropathy (DN) is a unique degenerative condition affecting the peripheral nervous system, specifically focusing on sensory and autonomic axons initially, followed by a lesser impact on motor axons [1]. Hyperalgesia, or excessive sensitivity to stimuli, and allodynia, or nociceptive reactions to non-noxious stimuli, are the hallmarks of neuropathic pain. It usually starts proximally from the hands and feet and proceeds in a stocking-glove pattern of scorching pain, paresthesia, and numbness. Neuropathic pain can emerge from various pathological conditions and circumstances, such as viral infections, metabolic irregularities, and autoimmune disorders that impact the central nervous system (CNS) [8]. Neuropathic pain deteriorates the overall subjective well-being of the patients suffering from DM [5].

To gain a deeper understanding of non-pharmacological interventions for managing neuropathic pain in individuals with diabetes mellitus (DM), it's essential to first grasp the pathophysiology of the disease and the mechanisms of action involved in pharmacological management. After we understand this concept, we will have a clear idea of how non-pharmacological management is more useful and efficient to relieve the pain of patients suffering from DPN.

Lesions that affect the somatosensory nerve system's structure as well as operation constitute the primary cause of pain associated with neuropathic conditions. It is characterized by spontaneous pain and exaggerated responses to both painful and non-painful stimuli. Maladaptive plasticity of the nociceptive system, which encompasses a range of neurological alterations, underlies this condition. Complex pain phenotypes arise from multiple changes distributed throughout the neural system. The anomalous production of action potentials, the loss of connections between synaptic cells, the development of new synaptic circuits, the acceleration and a lack of inhibition of synaptic transmission, and the interactions between the immune system and the nervous system are some of these alterations [9].

The pharmacological management of DPN is based on the severity of the disease [10].

Selecting medication for a specific patient is greatly influenced by various factors, such as the likelihood of side effects, managing concurrent conditions like depression or sleep disturbances, potential drug interactions, overdose or abuse risks, and cost. This is because recent evidence doesn't definitively rank medications based on efficacy. According to every guideline, a patient's specific pharmaceutical selections shall take in consideration all these aspects [11]. However, a study conducted by the International Association for the Study of Pain Neuropathic Pain Special Interest Group has outlined potential treatment approaches for neuropathic pain [12]. Figure 4.1 represents the hierarchy of pharmacological drugs used in the management of DPN. These medicines block the pain gate channels either by stopping the voltage-gated channels from binding to the calcium receptors or by blocking the neurotransmitters. This way the voltage-gated channels do not generate the action potential that would further generate the noxious stimulation that causes the pain sensation in patients [13].

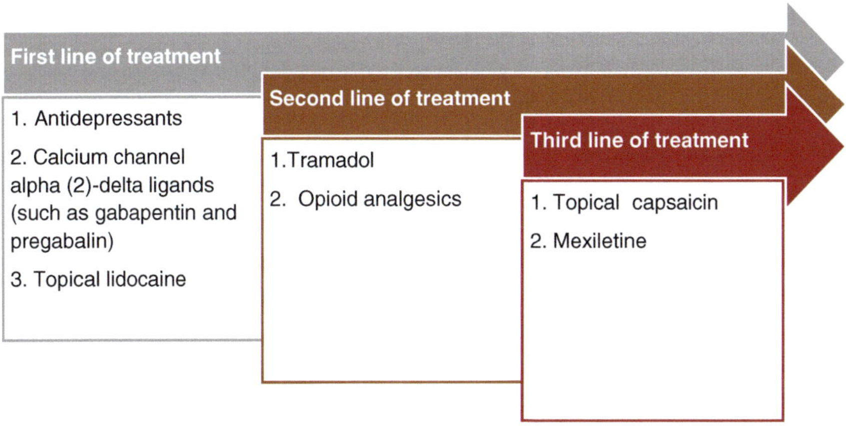

Fig. 4.1 The hierarchy of pharmacological management of DPN

Although these management strategies have their share of side effects, hence there is a demand to either adjunct these interventions with the non-pharmacological treatment methods or completely rely on non-pharmacological treatment methods.

4.3 Non-pharmacological Pain Interventions

Approximately, 8% of adult humans suffer from neuropathic pain, a complicated and varied illness that places a heavy strain on the patient and the healthcare system [14]. There is an urgent need to address the treatment gap for individuals experiencing diabetic peripheral neuropathy, as they often receive inadequate relief from conventional treatment methods. Researchers prove that non-pharmacological therapies be employed in DPN, mostly as an addition to pharmacological treatment [15]. DPN has a remarkably high illness burden, thus a growing need for innovative therapeutic management strategies that can be used either alone or in conjunction with existing treatments [16]. The non-pharmacological interventions for the management of painful diabetes neuropathy are the need of the hour to reduce the pain in people suffering from diabetes neuropathy [17]. Figure 4.2 represents a flowchart for various non-pharmacological management strategies that are based on evidence and can be used as a treatment of diabetes peripheral neuropathy. In the later section of this chapter, we will discuss these interventions in detail.

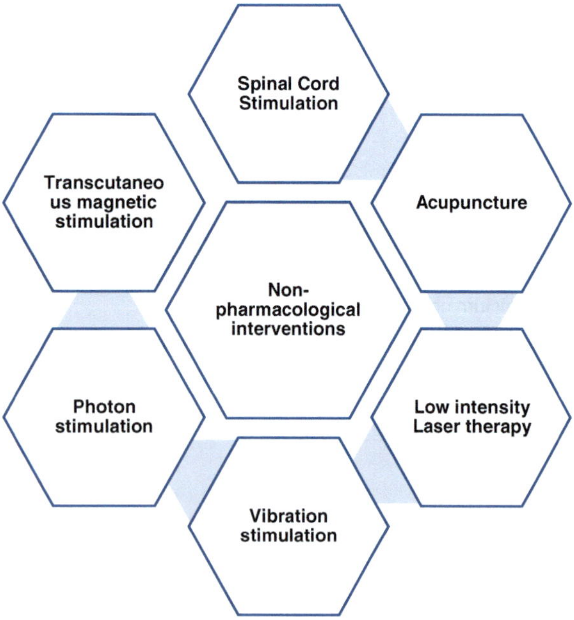

Fig. 4.2 The flow chart for non-pharmacological pain interventions

4.3.1 Spinal Cord Stimulation

The Pain Gate Theory—which will be discussed in the next section—underpins the mechanism of spinal cord stimulation (SCS), it has demonstrated a great deal of efficacy in reducing pain in individuals with severe neuropathic pain. The neurophysiology of spinal cord stimulation mechanism is idiopathic. Evidence depicts that both paresthesia-free and tonic SCS has great results in providing significant clinical analgesia [8].

An increasing amount of analysis has been documented in the literature in the past few decades that indicates spinal cord stimulation is an effective and risk-free therapy for diabetic peripheral neuropathy (DPN). As stated earlier, there is a potential gap in the treatment of DPN that much be addressed. Recent evidence shows that neuromodulation in combination with SCS has the potential to fill this gap in conservative treatment methodologies for the effective treatment of DPN pain [18]. The mechanism for modulating the nervous system is often a trade-off among location specificity, encroaching, and patient acceptability [19]. Although the precise mechanism underpinning tonic spinal cord stimulation (SCS) is still unknown, evidence points to the fact that SCS acts both at the spinal and supraspinal levels. Recently, new physiological targets for excitation and innovative SCS models have been proposed to bridge the gap between the current level of pain relief achievable with Tonic SCS and the desired pain relief. We shall study the mechanism in detail in later sections of the chapter.

4.3.1.1 How Does SCS Work?

The idea for SCS originated directly from the principle of gate control [20]. The "gate control theory" argued that the "spinal gate," situated in the posterior segment of the spinal cord, could be closed antidromically through the non-nociceptive Aβ fibers in the dorsal columns. Additionally, paresthesia or aberrant tingling sensations were experienced in the corresponding innervated location of the stimulated fibers upon orthodromic stimulation of the Aβ fibers in the back columns [21]. During the implantation of the SCS lead, the doctor ensures that these paraesthesia's cover the painful location. Based to the gate control theory, interneurons with inhibitory properties found in the higher laminae within the posterior horn close the "spinal gate". When these inhibitory interneurons are antidromically stimulated by spinal cord stimulation (SCS), they produce gamma-aminobutyric acid (GABA) to modulate the nociceptive signal [22]. Furthermore, research on rodents—basically rats—with ongoing neuropathic pain has shown that SCS lowers the back horn's internalized GABA immunoreactivity. The spinal posterior horn's extracellular GABA levels rise in tandem during the injection of SCS in chronic neuropathic rats. Therefore, one of the key components of the mechanisms behind SCS might be increased GABA release in the posterior horn of spinal cord. Therefore, presynaptic GABAB-mediated suppression of the connection between nociceptive afferents and the second-order neurons in the spinal posterior horn is a critical step in the process that allows tonic SCS. Nevertheless, postsynaptic GABAergic modulation via GABAA receptors when combined with K^+/Cl^- cotransporter 2 (KCC2) transcription are additionally involved in neuropathic pain and the process underlying SCS [21].

Rat models, such as the partial sciatic nerve ligation model (PSNL), have been employed in a majority of research on the impact of SCS. The electrodes are carefully inserted into the spinal space above the spinal dura mater. The posterior columns of the spinal cord are subsequently energized electrically using an external stimulation device or a removable pulse generator. The typical range of tonic SCS settings is 30–80 Hz, with wave widths of 100–500 μs and an amplitude that is greater than the sensory threshold [22].

Furthermore, various studies have used adjuvant stem cell therapy to treat refractory severe diabetic peripheral neuropathy [23]. The findings have demonstrated a notable decrease in pain intensity scores, which has been sustained for a minimum of 6 months. Now, let's talk about the side effects of SCS. It has some side effects, like postimplantation infections and subdural hematoma. The subdural hematoma may be due to dural puncture which may be life-threatening [24]. The incidence of patient death is rare.

4.3.1.2 How to Use SCS?

To understand more about SCS and its benefits, we have to know how we can use it. The SCS consists of two components: the implantable pulse generator (IPG) and the electrodes. These electrodes are also known as leads. SCS works by changing pulse-width modulation as it reduces the hyperexcitability of neurons by altering the local neurochemistry within dorsal horns using these implantable electrodes [25].

Most of the time, an external pulse generator is used to test the electrode for a week after it is percutaneously implanted using an epidural needle. Using a functional scale tailored to them, patients continuously document the degree of their discomfort and their capacity to carry out self-selected tasks during this time. If degenerative changes prevent the electrode from being inserted by an epidural needle, a neurosurgeon may also implant the electrode using a microsurgical method. Working together with the neurosurgery department is also crucial for handling any major side effects, even if these are quite uncommon [8].

The patient can select from a variety of stimulation programs using a portable device. The pulse generator will typically last for several years before needing to be replaced, but if power consumption is extremely high, installing a rechargeable pulse generator may be worth considering. Intermittent stimulation programs can extend the pulse generator's lifespan. The majority of more recent stimulation systems are MRI compatible, albeit certain scanner kinds and procedures could be needed [14]. Figure 4.3 depicts how spinal cord stimulator system operates.

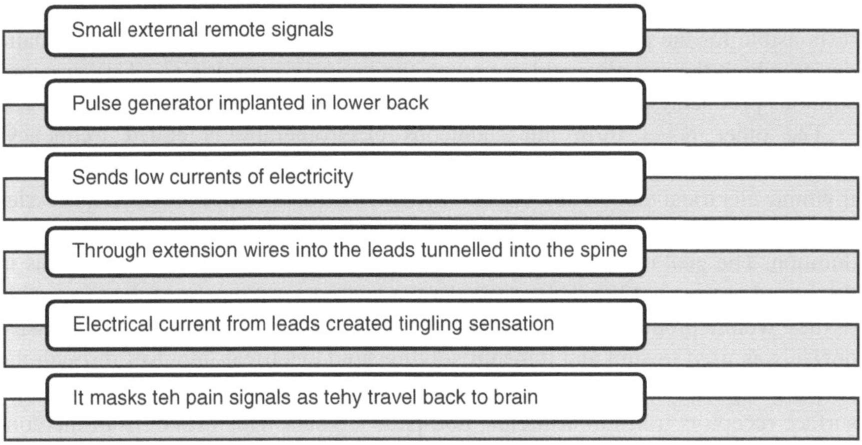

Fig. 4.3 Depicts how the spinal cord stimulator system operates

4.3.1.3 Complication of SCS

After the placement of percutaneous electrodes, SCS is a non-invasive procedure with a minimal chance of major side effects. Electrode breakage and migration are the most common problems [21].

4.3.2 Transcutaneous Electrical and Electromagnetic Stimulation

Recently, there is surge in studies using non-invasive neuromodulation (NINM) selectively on the oversight of diabetic peripheral neuropathic pain management. Peripheral and central neurostimulation comprise the further division of the NINM. Central neurostimulation is the most extensively researched form of neurostimulation and it comprises of repetitive transcranial magnetic stimulation (tDCS), the transcutaneous electrical neural stimulation (TENS) which is the most popular peripheral NINM technique and repetitive transcranial magnetic stimulation (rTMS) [26].

rTMS employs magnetic fields to cause electrical changes in brain activity, while tDCS works by using two electrodes over the scalp to give a subthreshold current from anode to cathode. TENS works on a similar concept; it basically alters the polarity of peripheral nerve membranes using an electrical current [27]. The basis for TENS is the pain gate theory, which was put forth by Melzack and Wall and is based on the neuromatrix theory of pain [20]. We have already studies in detail about the pain gate theory in the SCS section. Although, all are very well aware that TENS alters the perception of pain by altering maladaptive plasticity, thereby diminishing pain, and reinstating equilibrium in the regulation of inhibitory endogenous pain pathways [28]. In simple terms, the lateral spinothalamic tract is responsible for the pain sensation in our body. TENS reverses the signals of pain, due to which the signals could not reach the brain and we don't feel the noxious stimulus producing pain.

The other novel form transcutaneous electrotherapy is called frequency-modulated electromagnetic neural stimulation. The underlying concept of frequency rhythmic electrical modulation system (FREMS) involves the application of a series of voltage-controlled, regulated electrical stimuli, varying in pulse frequency and duration. The goal of this progressive change is to induce membrane potentials in the intended tissues [29]. This method was devised on the premise that excitable tissues would produce composite motor action potentials when a non-invasive device was used to sum and transmit subthreshold electrical impulses through the skin near a motor nerve. The core concept behind scrambler therapy is that C fiber surface receptors transmit artificial "non-pain" signals. This differs from the conventional electrical excitation of Aβ fibers, as seen with TENS, which aims to induce paresthesia and/or inhibit nerve fiber stimulation to induce an analgesic effect [30].

Research has demonstrated that additional static magnetic field therapy leads to significant reduction in pain brought on by exercise that is brought on by diabetic polyneuropathy.

Another electrophysical treatment is called interferential therapy, which uses two or four electrodes to apply electrical stimulation to the painful location at frequencies ranging from 1 to 1500 Hz. Long-wave diathermy at low power has its own benefits. It reduces the intensity of pain, but at contrary the long-wave diathermy at high power is less beneficial [31].

The transcutaneous electric and electromagnetic stimulation are proven to be highly efficient non-pharmacological intervention for DPN management.

4.3.3 Photon Stimulation

Both photo biomodulation and infrared light therapy are words used to describe photon stimulation, however they differ in wavelength. Photo biomodulation has the potential to enhance cellular metabolism and expedite cell and tissue healing [32]. The mechanism of action of photon stimulation is quite interesting to understand. The photon stimulation utilizes cytochrome c-oxidase (COX) and nitric oxide (NO). Research conducted at cellular level depict that the COX facilitates the absorption of light meanwhile NO works by inhibition of respiration by combining with the COX. So, the photon stimulation basically actions by making the bond between the COX and NO which further leads to segregation and disinhibition of mitochondria [33]. This leads to the stimulation of cytochromes present in the mitochondria which further initiates secondary signaling in the cells creating pathways for increased cellular healing and activity [34].

Low-intensity laser therapy is a safe non-pharmacological treatment approach with almost no side effects. Soon, it has the possibility to be a modality of choice in the care of patients with diabetic neuropathy [35]. Further studies are recommended to standardize the parameters of this novel treatment approach for DPN patients. The principle of low-intensity laser therapy (LILT) works on photochemical modulation. It means that at optimal energy densities and wavelengths, there is a change in biochemical triggers. This minimally invasive technique is not only a novel technique but also it can only deliver monochromatic light in the near-infrared to far-infrared region of the spectrum having a wavelength in 630–1000 nm range. After that, it makes use of supplementary photon stimulation to manage the PNP caused on by diabetic polyneuropathy of the lower extremities. Patients who underwent photon stimulation experienced improvement in sensation, social and mental functioning, and enhanced overall quality of life [5]. A plausible explanation for the decreased pain could be attributed to enhanced peripheral microcirculation. One potential explanation is that low-level laser therapy triggers the circulation's production of cytokines and growth hormones, which cause the vessels to dilate and new capillaries to develop. Literature depicts that exposure to He-Ne lasers causes the release of cytokines, which are essential for cell signaling, including IL-1α, IL-2, IFN-γ, and TNF-α. Increased ATP production by mitochondria and increased cellular oxygen demand by nerve regeneration are one of the potential causes of the pain reduction [36].

This concludes that photon stimulation is beneficial for as a non-pharmacological intervention in the management of DPN.

4.3.4 Vibration Stimulation

Vibratory stimulation (VS) is one of the non-pharmacological interventions that can have a possible implication in the treatment of DPN. Vibration stimulations works on the principle of neuromuscular activation and stimulation of the function of skeletal muscles. It is applied to the whole body or a specific part of the body that is painful with the help of a device. The device generates multiple pulses, leading to the enhancement of neuromuscular activation and skeletal muscle function, likely achieved by muscle tuning. In general, whole-body vibration (WBV) can be transmitted passively to the lower limbs in a particular position. In order to promote circulation, the patient half-squats while standing on a vibrating platform [37]. The glycemic profile is marginally improved by VS; however, the quality of the evidence is questionable. Although there is no data to support these results, people with DPN appear to have improved neuropathic pain and balance following WBV treatments. Future research is probably going to alter the estimated effect, which means that the current usage of WBV in DPN patients for neuropathic pain relief, balance enhancement, and plantar tactile sensitivity is not supported much [11].

4.3.5 Acupuncture

Acupuncture is a least intrusive procedure that involves minimal damage into body cavity. It originated from traditional Chinese medicine, and it works on the principle of meridian theory [38]. The meridian theory works on facts and experiments. The meridians are not characterized on anatomical structures formally, but there are acupoints. These acupoints are like road maps. It is hypothesized that acupuncture increases local microcirculation, which improves the neural tissue's supply to some extent [39]. There is less evidence that acupuncture is beneficial for the management of DPN, but still it is one of the most popular non-pharmacological interventions used nowadays.

4.3.6 Neurofeedback

Neurofeedback is an intervention of learning which could be used as a non-medicinal treatment intervention. It is basically the conscious management of brain waves and monitoring their development. Brain activity is the focus of a non-invasive therapy called neurofeedback (NF). Patients can actively alter their brain activities in ways that may improve their comfort and health with biofeedback, which gives them access to information about their brain activity [40]. This can be achieved by active learning.

NF can be carried out by employing functional magnetic resonance imaging (fMRI) or brain activity as known as electroencephalography (EEG). Because EEG biofeedback equipment is more widely available and less expensive, the EEG method is utilized far more frequently. When using EEG-based neural feedback, the patient has one or more electrodes inserted on their scalp to detect the oscillatory activity's amplitude, or "power," over several frequency bandwidths. In the cortex, directly below the electrode, the raw electrical signal is the collective activity of millions of neurons [41]. A portion of the electrical brain activity is evaluated and sent back to the patient. The basis of fMRI-based neurofeedback is the blood oxygen level dependent (BOLD) areas of focus in the brain that exhibit increased activity, whereas EEG-based NF typically targets modifications in the power of activity in particular oscillation bandwidths [42]. Numerous health conditions, such as pain management, sleep disorders, and traumatic brain injuries have been effectively treated with it when combined with prescription drugs. The conceptualization of neurofeedback is quite interesting to understand.

Whether NF is performed using fMRI or EEG, the patient receives feedback on the measured alterations in brain activity. Sometimes, but not usually, a game is used to deliver feedback. When a patient modifies the targeted brain activity (e.g., increases alpha power recorded over the sensory cortex), a program may enable the patient to "fly" a plane. If the targeted brain activity is moving in the direction of the training criteria set by the therapist, the plane will fly smoothly; if it is moving in a different direction, the plane may crash or have other problems. Through operant conditioning, this feedback affects the patient's brain activity and gradually teaches it to alter. It's crucial to remember that while the most famous NF therapies depend on the theory of operant conditioning, certain NF types use alternative theories. Furthermore, NF treatment frequently takes a while to cause changes in brain activity; a full course of NF treatment typically consists of 15–50 sessions lasting 20–40 min each [42].

Evidence shows that neurofeedback is a highly effective non-pharmacological management of DPN. It alters the brain activity and helps patients cope up with the pain. Thus, this intervention can be used for individuals of any age. Neurofeedback is one of the most motivating and interesting ways for the management of DPN pain.

4.4 Conclusion

This chapter concludes that the non-pharmacological interventions may be a game-changing intervention that may cure the pain of patients suffering with diabetes peripheral neuropathy.

It may be used alone or in conjunction with the pharmacological interventions in the management of DPN.

References

1. Feldman EL, Callaghan BC, Pop-Busui R, Zochodne DW, Wright DE, Bennett DL, Bril V, Russell JW, Viswanathan V. Diabetic neuropathy. Nat Rev Dis Primers. 2019;5(1):41. https://doi.org/10.1038/s41572-019-0092-1.
2. Deshpande AD, Harris-Hayes M, Schootman M. Epidemiology of diabetes and diabetes-related complications. Phys Ther. 2008;88(11):1254–64.
3. American Diabetes Association. Diagnosis and classification of diabetes mellitus. Diabetes Care. 2010;33(Suppl 1):S62–9. https://doi.org/10.2337/dc10-S062. Erratum in: Diabetes Care. 2010 Apr;33(4):e57.
4. Kharroubi AT, Darwish HM. Diabetes mellitus: tThe epidemic of the century. World J Diabetes. 2015;6(6):850–67.
5. Saraf A, Goyal M, Vileikyte L, Ateef M, Samuel AJ. Neuropathy-and foot-ulcer specific quality of life instrument (NeuroQoL): translation, cross-cultural adaptation, and content validation in Hindi. Foot Ankle Surg. 2023;29(2):105–10. https://doi.org/10.1016/j.fas.2022.11.003.
6. Bhutani J, Bhutani S. Worldwide burden of diabetes. Indian J Endocrinol Metab. 2014;18(6):868–70.
7. Jang HN, Oh TJ. Pharmacological and nonpharmacological treatments for painful diabetic peripheral neuropathy. Diabetes Metab J. 2023;47(6):743–56. https://doi.org/10.4093/dmj.2023.0018.
8. Finnerup NB, Kuner R, Jensen TS. Neuropathic pain: from mechanisms to treatment. Physiol Rev. 2021;101(1):259–301.
9. Becerra L, Morris S, Bazes S, Gostic R, Sherman S, Gostic J, et al. Trigeminal neuropathic pain alters responses in CNS circuits to mechanical (brush) and thermal (cold and heat) stimuli. J Neurosci. 2006;26(42):10646–57.

10. Abbafati C, Abbas KM, Abbasi-Kangevari M, Abd-Allah F, Abdelalim A, Abdollahi M, et al. Global burden of 369 diseases and injuries in 204 countries and territories, 1990–2019: a systematic analysis for the Global Burden of Disease Study 2019. Lancet. 2020;396(10258):1204–22.
11. Moisset X, Bouhassira D, Avez Couturier J, Alchaar H, Conradi S, Delmotte MH, et al. Pharmacological and non-pharmacological treatments for neuropathic pain: systematic review and French recommendations. Rev Neurol (Paris). 2020;176(5):325–52.
12. O'Connor AB, Dworkin RH. Treatment of neuropathic pain: an overview of recent guidelines. Am J Med. 2009;122(Suppl 10):S22–32. https://doi.org/10.1016/j.amjmed.2009.04.007.
13. Bates D, Carsten Schultheis B, Hanes MC, Jolly SM, Chakravarthy KV, Deer TR, et al. A comprehensive algorithm for management of neuropathic pain. Pain Med. 2019;20(Suppl 1):S2–S12. https://doi.org/10.1093/pm/pnz075.
14. Bernetti A, Agostini F, de Sire A, Mangone M, Tognolo L, Di Cesare A, Ruiu P, Paolucci T, Invernizzi M, Paoloni M. Neuropathic pain and rehabilitation: a systematic review of international guidelines. Diagnostics (Basel). 2021;11(1):74. https://doi.org/10.3390/diagnostics11010074.
15. Jahantigh Akbari N, Hosseinifar M, Naimi SS, Mikaili S, Rahbar S. The efficacy of physiotherapy interventions in mitigating the symptoms and complications of diabetic peripheral neuropathy: a systematic review. J Diabetes Metab Disord. 2020;19(2):1995–2004. https://doi.org/10.1007/s40200-020-00652-8.
16. Saatmann N, Zaharia OP, Loenneke JP, Roden M, Pesta DH. Effects of blood flow restriction exercise and possible applications in type 2 diabetes. Trends Endocrinol Metab. 2021;32(2):106–17. https://doi.org/10.1016/j.tem.2020.11.010.
17. Liampas A, Rekatsina M, Vadalouca A, Paladini A, Varrassi G, Zis P. Non-pharmacological management of painful peripheral neuropathies: a systematic review. Adv Ther. 2020;37(10):4096–106. https://doi.org/10.1007/s12325-020-01462-3.
18. Denison T, Morrell MJ. Neuromodulation in 2035 the neurology future forecasting series. Neurology. 2022;98(2):65–72.
19. Henson JV, Varhabhatla NC, Bebic Z, Kaye AD, Yong RJ, Urman RD, et al. Spinal cord stimulation for painful diabetic peripheral neuropathy: a systematic review. Pain Ther. 2021;10(2):895–908. https://doi.org/10.1007/s40122-021-00282-9.
20. Melzack R, Wall PD. Pain mechanisms: a new theory. Science. 1965;150:971–9. https://doi.org/10.1126/science.150.3699.971.
21. Meyerson BA, Linderoth B. Mode of action of spinal cord stimulation in neuropathic pain. J Pain Symptom Manag. 2006;31(Suppl 4):S6–12. https://doi.org/10.1016/j.jpainsymman.2005.12.009.
22. Smits H, van Kleef M, Holsheimer J, Joosten EA. Experimental spinal cord stimulation and neuropathic pain: mechanism of action, technical aspects, and effectiveness. Pain Pract. 2013;13(2):154–68. https://doi.org/10.1111/j.1533-2500.2012.00579.x.
23. Scholz J, Finnerup NB, Attal N, Aziz Q, Baron R, Bennett MI, et al. The IASP classification of chronic pain for ICD-11: chronic neuropathic pain. Pain. 2019;160(1):53–9. https://doi.org/10.1097/j.pain.0000000000001365.
24. Duarte RV, Andronis L, Lenders MWPM, de Vos CC. Quality of life increases in patients with painful diabetic neuropathy following treatment with spinal cord stimulation. Qual Life Res. 2016;25(7):1771–7. https://doi.org/10.1007/s11136-015-1211-4.
25. Joosten EA, Franken G. Spinal cord stimulation in chronic neuropathic pain: mechanisms of action, new locations, new paradigms. Pain. 2020;161 Suppl 1(1):S104–13. https://doi.org/10.1097/j.pain.0000000000001854.
26. Zeng H, Pacheco-Barrios K, Cao Y, Li Y, Zhang J, Yang C, Fregni F. Non-invasive neuromodulation effects on painful diabetic peripheral neuropathy: a systematic review and meta-analysis. Sci Rep. 2020;10(1):19184. https://doi.org/10.1038/s41598-020-75922-9.
27. Mendell LM. Constructing and deconstructing the gate theory of pain. Pain. 2014;155(2):210–6. https://doi.org/10.1016/j.pain.2013.12.010.
28. Costigan M, Scholz J, Woolf CJ. Neuropathic pain: a maladaptive response of the nervous system to damage. Annu Rev Neurosci. 2009;32:1–32. https://doi.org/10.1146/annurev.neuro.051508.135531.

29. Majeedkutty NA, Jabbar MA, Sreenivasulu S. Physical therapy for diabetic peripheral neuropathy: a narrative review. Disabil CBR Incl Dev. 2019;30(1):112–25.
30. Petersen T, Laslett M, Juhl C. Clinical classification in low back pain: best-evidence diagnostic rules based on systematic reviews. BMC Musculoskelet Disord. 2017;18(1):188. https://doi.org/10.1186/s12891-017-1549-6.
31. Klinger R, Stuhlreyer J, Schwartz M, Schmitz J, Colloca L. Clinical use of placebo effects in patients with pain disorders. Int Rev Neurobiol. 2018;139:107–28. https://doi.org/10.1016/bs.irn.2018.07.015.
32. Zinman LH, Ngo M, Ng ET, Nwe KT, Gogov S, Bril V. Low-intensity laser therapy for painful symptoms of diabetic sensorimotor polyneuropathy: a controlled trial. Diabetes Care. 2004;27(4):921–4. https://doi.org/10.2337/diacare.27.4.921.
33. Ebadi SA, Tabeie F, Tavakoli S, Khalili S. Effects of photobiomodulation with two wavelengths of 630 and 810 nm on diabetic neuropathy. J Lasers Med Sci. 2023;14:e22. https://doi.org/10.34172/jlms.2023.22.
34. Swislocki A, Orth M, Bales M, Weisshaupt J, West C, Edrington J, et al. A randomized clinical trial of the effectiveness of photon stimulation on pain, sensation, and quality of life in patients with diabetic peripheral neuropathy. J Pain Symptom Manag. 2010;39(1):88–99.
35. Khamseh ME, Kazemikho N, Aghili R, Forough B, Lajevardi M, Hashem Dabaghian F, Goushegir A, Malek M. Diabetic distal symmetric polyneuropathy: effect of low-intensity laser therapy. Lasers Med Sci. 2011;26(6):831–5. https://doi.org/10.1007/s10103-011-0977-z.
36. Hashmi JT, Huang YY, Osmani BZ, Sharma SK, Naeser MA, Hamblin MR. Role of low-level laser therapy in neurorehabilitation. PM R. 2010;2(12):S292–305. https://doi.org/10.1016/j.pmrj.2010.10.013.
37. Robinson CC, Barreto RPG, Plentz RDM. Effects of whole body vibration in individuals with diabetic peripheral neuropathy: a systematic review. J Musculoskelet Neuronal Interact. 2018;18(3):382–8.
38. Dietzel J, Habermann IV, Hörder S, Hahn K, Meyer-Hamme G, Ortiz M, et al. Acupuncture in patients with diabetic peripheral neuropathy-related complaints: a randomized controlled clinical trial. J Clin Med. 2023;12(6):2103. https://doi.org/10.3390/jcm12062103.
39. Yu B, Li M, Huang H, Ma S, Huang K, Zhong Z, Yu S, Zhang L. Acupuncture treatment of diabetic peripheral neuropathy: an overview of systematic reviews. J Clin Pharm Ther. 2021;46(3):585–98. https://doi.org/10.1111/jcpt.13351.
40. Apkarian AV, Hashmi JA, Baliki MN. Pain and the brain: specificity and plasticity of the brain in clinical chronic pain. Pain. 2011;152(Suppl 3):S49–64. https://doi.org/10.1016/j.pain.2010.11.010.
41. Hassan MA, Fraser M, Conway BA, Allan DB, Vuckovic A. The mechanism of neurofeedback training for treatment of central neuropathic pain in paraplegia: a pilot study. BMC Neurol. 2015;15(1):200. https://doi.org/10.1186/s12883-015-0445-7.
42. Roy R, de la Vega R, Jensen MP, Miró J. Neurofeedback for pain management: a systematic review. Front Neurosci. 2020;14:671. https://doi.org/10.3389/fnins.2020.00671.

Chapter 5
Exercise Therapy Interventions for DPN

Muskan and Shweta Sharma

Contents

Muskan (✉)
Physiotherapy, SGT University, Gurugram, Haryana, India

S. Sharma
MM Institute of Physiotherapy & Rehabilitation, Maharishi Markandeshwar (Deemed to be University), Ambala, Haryana, India

© The Author(s), under exclusive license to Springer Nature Singapore Pte Ltd. 2024
M. Goyal, K. Goyal (eds.), *Rehabilitation in Diabetic Peripheral Neuropathy*,
https://doi.org/10.1007/978-981-97-9290-0_5

5.1 Introduction

The global number of diabetics is expected to double from 2000 to 366 million by 2030, with diabetes mellitus being a major public health concern [1]. By 2045, there will be 693 million diabetics worldwide, with diabetic peripheral neuropathy (DPN) being the most prevalent and serious microvascular consequence [2]. DPN is linked to poor glycemic management, long-term diabetes, hyperlipidemia, higher albumin excretion rates, and obesity [3–7].

5.2 Exercise-Based Interventions

Patients with diabetes often experience poor muscle coordination and DPN, leading to gait abnormalities, postural instability, and falls. Understanding how diabetic polyneuropathy and vestibular system dysfunction affect falls is crucial for fall prevention and maintaining postural stability [8].

Exercise including weightlifting was once thought to be dangerous for those with diabetic nephropathy (DPN). However, research has shown that weight-bearing therapies, such as aerobic activities, strengthening, flexibility, and progressive balancing, can increase walking distance and average daily step count without increasing adverse events. El-Refay and Ali discovered that an 8-week exercise regimen focusing on flexibility, range of motion, muscle growth, and gait training increased walking speed, reduced step time, and improved ankle range of motion during the gait's stance phase [9] (Fig. 5.1). Kanchana Samut and Pensri found that peak plantar pressure at the medial forefoot decreased in the exercise group but not in the control group. These findings suggest that weight-bearing exercise could be an effective method for DPN patients to enhance their foot-ankle complex and reduce plantar pressure [10]. In diabetics with or without peripheral neuropathy, 8–12 weeks of physical exercise increases the conduction velocity of the motor tibial, peroneal, and sensory sural nerves [11].

5.2.1 ADA (American Diabetics Association) Precautionary Guidelines for Exercise with DPN [12] (Fig. 5.2)

1. Start with low-impact exercise: To prevent overexertion and injury, people with DPN should begin with low-intensity activities and progressively increase the intensity and duration.
2. Check Blood Sugar Levels: Because exercise elevates blood sugar levels, diabetics must monitor their glucose levels both before and after exercise.

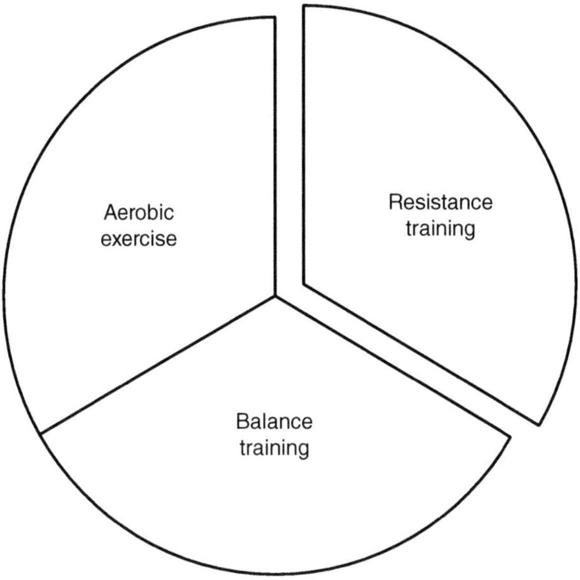

Fig. 5.1 Elements of exercise. (Source: Self)

3. Foot Care: Wearing the right shoes is crucial to keeping your feet safe. Checking your feet every day can help prevent problems.
4. Keep Yourself Hydrated: Staying properly hydrated is crucial, particularly for those with diabetes who may have altered thirst feelings.

5.3 Aerobic Exercise Training

A well-researched exercise technique is aerobic exercise, which entails rhythmic, vigorous motions over an extended period. It is associated with improved respiratory health and reduces the overall mortality from heart disease. Research has shown that aerobic exercise improves a person with type 2 diabetes's body composition, maximum intake of oxygen, and glucose metabolism. Chronic physical activity can also result in significant reductions in systolic and diastolic blood pressure, body fat percentage terms, triglycerides, low-density lipoproteins, fasting blood glucose, HbA1c, and triglycerides. For example in a research, subjects engaged in three times a week, 16 weeks of closely monitored aerobic exercise under the guidance of medical experts or students certified in CPR. The monitoring of adherence to the research protocol involved observation, instruction, and routine assessment of exercise logs. Heart rate was recorded before, during, and after each session, ranging in

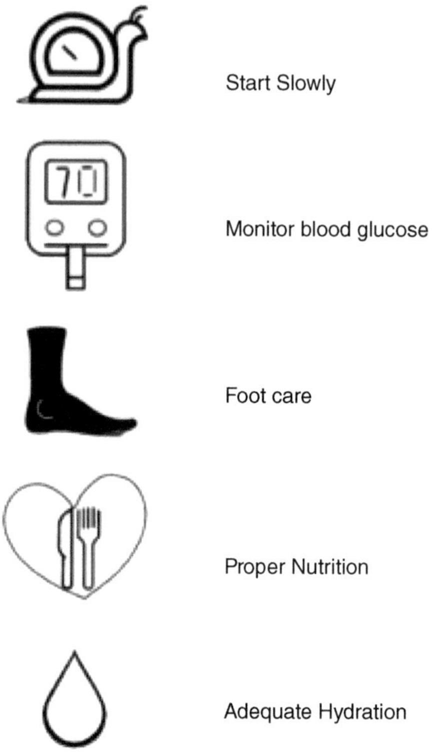

Fig. 5.2 Guidelines for exercise. (Source: https://www.istockphoto.com/vector/slow-vector-icon-slow-editable-stroke-slow-linear-symbol-for-use-on-web-and-mobile-gm1250143832-364528044; https://www.vecteezy.com/vector-art/2096328-glucose-monitor-icon-glucometer-line-vector-eps; https://www.vecteezy.com/vector-art/28739286-restaurant-line-icon-isolated-on-white-background-fork-spoon-and-plate-icon)

duration from 30 to 50 min. Every session began and ended with a blood pressure check. If resting blood pressure was increased to values close to stage 2 hypertension, it was tested every 10–15 min while exercising. During the graded maximal exercise test, each person's heart rate response was used to determine the appropriate aerobic activity intensity [13] (Fig. 5.3).

People with Type 2 diabetes mellitus benefit from aerobic exercise because it enhances vascular endothelial function (T2DM). The vascular condition of people with type 2 diabetes and peripheral neuropathy due to diabetes (DPN) is not well-understood. Determining whether a 16-week aerobic exercise intervention might enhance vascular health in individuals with T2DM and DPN was, thus, the main goal of this secondary study. Examining the connection between variations in flow-mediated dilation (FMD) and the duration elapsed after DPN diagnosis was a secondary goal [14].

Aerobic exercise affected the anthropometric, hemodynamic, and metabolic profiles of people with type 2 diabetes. The findings indicated that blood glucose,

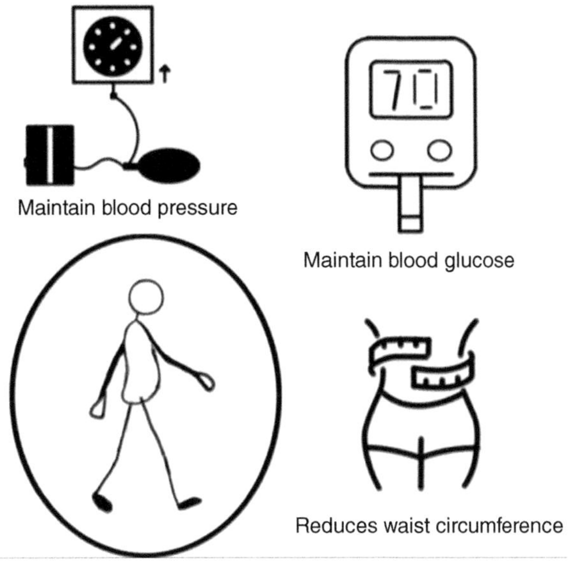

Fig. 5.3 Benefits of Aerobic training. (Source: https://www.vecteezy.com/vector-art/5724564-measurement-size-of-circumference-waist-with-tape-line-icon-slim-waistline-with-measure-tape-linear-pictogram-female-beauty-shape-concept-outline-icon-isolated-vector-illustration; https://www.vecteezy.com/vector-art/2096328-glucose-monitor-icon-glucometer-line-vector-eps; https://www.flaticon.com/free-icon/blood-pressure-meter_10251156)

diastolic blood pressure, and waist circumference were all significantly decreased by moderate-intensity aerobic exercise performed three or more times per week. Therefore, diabetes type 2 patients benefit from regular, moderate-intensity aerobic exercise [15].

Participants can use various aerobic workout equipment, including elliptical trainers, treadmills, recumbent steppers, and cycle ergometers. Training session included the target HR duration and began with a 5–10-minute warm-up and cool-down [16].

Mindfulness training combined with aerobic exercise has a great therapeutic effect and is essential for enhancing neurological function and quality of life. It's a secure and useful form of therapy. Thus, the combination of mindfulness training with physical exercise ought to be promoted and put into practice [17].

5.3.1 Aerobic Exercise and Sensorimotor Function

Studies have indicated that heart rate (HR) measures for the prescription of moderate-to-intense aerobic exercise may be a useful strategy for reducing the symptoms of DPN in T2D patients. Research has shown that the probable mechanism for the ensuing benefits might be the manipulation of sorbitol levels. Increased intracellular sorbitol content has been shown to cause damage to Schwann cells, which may result in a neuronal environment that is hypoxic all the time [18].

Hyperglycemia can increase the generation of superoxide, which can cause vascular distensibility and endothelial dysfunction. For those with type 2 diabetes, aerobic exercise training can boost flow-mediated dilatation and thereby improve endothelial function. Because of increased nitric oxide synthesis and improved endothelial function, one adaptation to aerobic endurance training may have been the restoration of blood vessel compliance and the reversal of the low oxygen level associated with normal DPN development [19, 20].

Individuals with DPN are physically inactive due to neuropathic pain and reduced sensorimotor function; as such, they are prime candidate for aerobic exercise therapies. Perceived pain during varied daily tasks was significantly reduced after a 16-week supervised aerobic exercise program. Lower levels of protein kinase C and advanced glycation end products were thought to be the cause. Which are normally elevated in response to persistent hyperglycemia. After a 15-week high-intensity interval training exercise, Hamed and Raoof saw significant improvements in pain as judged by the Leeds Assessment of Neuropathic Symptoms and Signs Scale and significant reductions in fasting and 2-hour blood glucose levels [21].

5.3.2 Aerobic Exercise and Cardiovascular Physical Fitness

The risk of mortality from any reason is strongly correlated with cardiovascular health, and early mortality is significantly exacerbated by sedentary behavior. Diabetic peripheral neuropathy (DPN) and type 2 diabetes are associated with fatigue during everyday activities, which may lead to a reduction in cardiorespiratory fitness, a weakening of the muscles, and an increase in body fat.

When designing an aerobic fitness training program for individuals with diabetic peripheral neuropathy (DPN), additional complexity arises. Due to elevated blood pressure and cholesterol, people with diabetes are more vulnerable to heart attacks and strokes. Certain reactions to exercise can be blunted and the amount of work that can be done at a high intensity by certain heart disease drugs. Leading indicators of cardiovascular autonomic neuropathy include exercise intolerance, orthostatic hypotension, resting tachycardia, reduced heart rate variability, and other non-specific symptoms a common T2D consequence that is frequently overlooked. The risk of cardiovascular events and death is exacerbated by this autonomic dysfunction [22].

In research by Morrison et al., people with DPN did three aerobic exercise sessions a week for 12 weeks. They were divided into two groups: intense and moderate-intensity aerobic exercise. The findings revealed considerable improvements in insulin concentrations, glycated hemoglobin (Hba1c), and fasting blood glucose levels, but only modest increases in peak oxygen absorption. Along with these improvements in gait velocity, stride length, step length, and time spent in stance, participants also showed decreases in body fat [23].

VO2 peak significantly increased and total body fat decreased after 16 weeks of moderate-intensity aerobic activity, three times a week. Both the overall and physical exhaustion ratings showed improvements. Diabetes reduces exercise capacity and limits peak oxygen consumption because diabetics have peripheral vascular dysfunction and decreased heart responses during exercise.

According to preliminary data, aerobic exercise regularly for periods of at least 8 weeks, at both moderate and intense intensities, can lead to positive improvements in metabolic function and cardiorespiratory fitness. These enhancements may then promote greater engagement in regular exercise and enhance glycemic management [24].

5.4 Resistance Exercise Training

The popular technique of resistance exercise training is used to increase muscle growth, strength, power, and endurance. It is used to improve sports performance, health, and fitness through the gradual application of different resistive loads and training modes (Fig. 5.4). Research focuses on the potential benefits of exercising with resistance on capillary perfusion, synaptic drive, and control of glucose since these factors are important mediators of neuropathic muscle adaptation [25, 26].

When working with individuals who have diabetes or low glucose tolerance, it is recommended to begin with 1–3 sets of 10–15 repetitions at moderate intensities of 50–69% 1-RM for 8–10 exercises that target the complete body. It is recommended to work your way up to sets of 8–10 repetitions or 70–85% "vigorous" intensities. 1-RM [6].

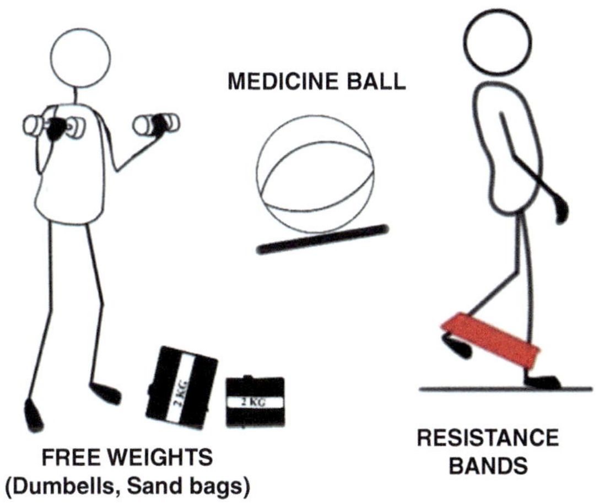

Fig. 5.4 Types of resistance equipment. (Source: Self)

5.4.1 Resistance Training and Glycemic Control

It has been shown that resistance training improves HbA1c and insulin sensitivity for people with Type 2 Diabetes (T2D), especially in the initial phases of the disease in those with less muscle mass index. Regular resistance training is especially helpful for senior citizens since sarcopenia, or the aging-related loss of muscle mass in the skeleton, increases the risk of diabetes and impaired glucose tolerance. Resistance training has been shown to enhance the body composition of older individuals by improving glucose disappearance rates and lowering hypoglycemia area-under-the-curve by 25–28% in tolerance to oral glucose tests [27].

5.4.2 Resistance Training and Microvascular Perfusion

Peripheral vascular dysfunction is common among diabetics, and it can get worse when diabetic peripheral nephropathy (DPN) occurs. In healthy individuals, long-term strength training can significantly reduce arterial stiffness. Improved nitric oxide generation can result in higher dilatation of blood vessels and improved blood flow during a 12-week resistance exercise program. In different feed stages, whole-body resistance exercise can also improve vascular conductance and leg blood flow [28].

5.4.3 Resistance Training and Neural Drive

People who have DPN are more likely to fall, and 60% of fall-related fatalities happen while a person is going downstairs. This is because age-related sarcopenia in older persons might worsen reduced muscular activation. It has been demonstrated that regular resistance training (RT) increases strength and power through age-neutral neuronal adaptations. By improving skeletal muscle fiber size, work efficiency, core strength, balance, stability, and work efficiency, RT programs can lower the risk of falls. Participants in a 16-week resistance training (RT) intervention performed leg extension, leg press, and ankle press exercises in three sets of 12 repetitions, with 1 min of rest in between. Results from the post-test revealed that during both stair climb and descent, the patients with DPN generated strength in their knee and ankle at a considerably faster pace [29–31].

5.4.4 Concurrent Aerobic and Resistance Exercise Training

As was already noted, the training intervention that is most frequently used in the scientific literature to examine the benefits of exercise on individuals with DPN is aerobic exercise. Conversely, little research has been done on the efficiency of resistance exercise training. Nonetheless, individuals with DPN have been investigated while using a combined aerobic and resistance exercise training strategy.

After completing a 10-week aerobic and strengthening exercise program, persons with diabetic peripheral neuropathy (DPN) reported reduced pain, improved nerve fiber branching, and symptom ratings. Following combination training, Nadi et al. saw improvements in sensory-motor function. Significant improvements were seen in DPN patients' lower limb numbness, discomfort, tingling, and weakness. Nonetheless, it was not shown that vitamin D administration significantly changed the electrophysiologic characteristics of peripheral sensory and motor nerves. The length of the intervention and the degree of peripheral nerve fiber damage determine whether neuropathy signs and symptoms can be reversed [32].

5.5 Balance and Proprioception-Based Exercise Training

In older individuals, damage to the motor and sensory neurons can cause sarcopenia, balance problems, and muscular atrophy. To address this issue, practitioners looked into therapeutic strategies that enhanced equilibrium. Studies have shown a significant reduction in body sway with eyes open and closed, as well as improvements in dynamic equilibrium scores from the Berg Balance Scale, Functional Reach Test, Timed Up and Go test, and 10-m walking time (Fig. 5.5).

Furthermore, a reduction in trunk repositioning mistakes in three different scenarios—eyes open stable surface, eyes closed stable surface, and eyes open foam—improves trunk proprioception [33] (Fig. 5.5).

People with DPN experience postural instability due to inaccurate proprioceptive signals from their lower extremities, which affects their ability to coordinate crucial reflexes and joint actions. Yoga-based therapies have been proposed as a substitute for conventional exercise therapy aimed at improving flexibility and balance. Yoga, much more so than traditional balance activities, was reported by Boslego et al. to dramatically enhance balance confidence and Berg Balance Scale scores in people with DPN [34]. A 12-week yoga training intervention was studied by Kanjirathingal

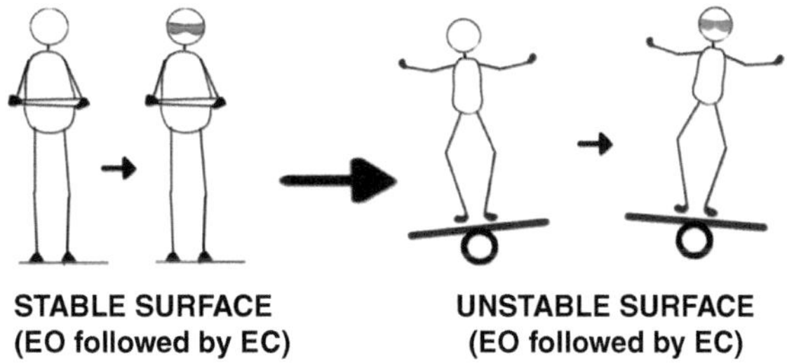

Fig. 5.5 Balance training. *EO* Eyes open, *EC* Eyes closed. (Source: Self)

et al., who found that the end measurements for strength and balance significantly increased. Greater reach lengths anteriorly, postero-laterally, and postero-medially were seen in the Star excursion balancing test [35].

Dynamic balance performance and single-limb stance time can both be markedly enhanced by yoga intervention. The somatosensory system is targeted by the positions Vrikshasana, Utkatasana, Tadasana, Padhastasana, and Garudasana, which maintain the head, arm, and trunk within a small foundation while stimulating proprioceptors [35, 36].

Vestibular and somatosensory systems are challenged by Ardhachandrasanas, Natrajasana, Virabhadrasana I, II, and III. When yoga is used instead of traditional training, lower extremity strength improves by 30% more. This results from enhanced lower extremity muscular strength and endurance as well as the targeted stimulation of hip and core muscle areas, which are essential for maintaining balance. The hip extensors, knee extensors, and ankle plantar flexors are the three main lower extremity antigravity muscles that are engaged in these postures. In summary, yoga intervention has demonstrated encouraging outcomes in terms of enhancing lower extremity strength, dynamic balancing performance, and postures [37].

Another type of exercise that has been researched for its potential to help individuals with long-term medical and mental issues is tai chi, often known as tai chi chuan. For instance, 12 weeks, Ahn and Song arranged for 20 people with DPN to take part in two 1-hour tai chi sessions each week. The neuropathic overall symptom score, balance score, and glucose control all showed improvements [38].

For daily tasks including sitting, walking, and standing, balance must be maintained. By affecting the anticipatory postural response, which affects trunk control and muscle activation, Swiss ball training can aid with balance improvement. The postural disruption caused by the Swiss ball movement enables the trunk muscles to adapt and preserve stability. There is a significant rise in equilibrium as a result. Swiss ball exercises increase muscle mass, motor and sensory capacities for movement, and stride length, velocity, and cadence. Patients' range of motion increases with repeated usage of the Swiss ball training program, which significantly affects these outcomes. Therefore, using a Swiss ball for fitness training can assist persons with diabetic neuropathy become more mobile and balance [39].

The most promising clinical evidence for addressing balance impairment in DPN patients is the use of lower extremity strengthening exercises as an intervention. As of right now, there are insufficient high-quality studies with sound methodology and significant clinical results to back up the usage of vibrating insoles, monochromatic infrared radiation, or canes.The purpose of this study is to assess how well patients with diabetic peripheral neuropathy respond to interactive video game-based (IVGB) activities for balance training and rehabilitation. Because they are repetitious, traditional balancing exercise regimens like static posture maintenance are typically viewed as ugly. Patients' balance, movement, and overall quality of life have all improved with the help of line dancing and tai chi softball. Patients are encouraged to engage in training activities by the increased enjoyment and attractiveness of IVGB exercises [40].

Patients with DPN needed to learn how to coordinate their hip and distal joint motions and transfer their weight, which was facilitated by the ankle-reaching exercise. Without elevating their toes or heels, participants were asked to move their hips in the anterior–posterior (AP) direction to produce dorsiflexion/plantarflexion at the ankle. To complete a single cycle of the ankle-reaching challenge, the activity was repeated from the goal to the starting circle [41].

The American Diabetes Association recommends that persons with diabetic foot (DPN) train in both strength and balance. Sand can offer an unstable surface and resistance, extending the duration between contractions and increasing muscle activity. Previous studies on older individuals found that training on sandy surfaces improved proprioceptive perception, balance, balance capacity, and muscle activation. Exercise in the sand can assist DPN patients to improve their functional abilities, strength, and balance while minimizing their injury risk. Sand exercises, which incorporate resistance, balance, and muscle stretching stimulation, may improve foot function. For 12 weeks, barefoot training sessions were held three times a week in a heated 4 × 5 m sandbox [42].

Weight-bearing and foot-ankle therapy exercises have been shown to have positive benefits on people with diabetic peripheral neuropathy. The workouts focused on the ankle, metatarsophalangeal, medial, lateral, median, and dorsal plantar side muscle groups as well as the interphalangeal and ankle joints. Reduced plantar numbness, improved ankle range of motion in the sagittal plane, increased conductivity speed of the peroneal motor nerve and sural sensory nerve, expanded peripheral microvasculature, modified vascular function, and improved sensory and motor afferent function were among the results. Additionally, the calcaneal tendon's mechanical properties were enhanced. Additionally, research indicates that diabetes individuals may benefit from a straightforward, inexpensive, low-risk, and quickly improving treatment regimen that includes mini-trampolines and ankle therapeutic exercises [43].

5.6 Cutting Edge Tools for Assessment and Training Gait and Balance

5.6.1 FOotCAre (FOCA) Trial II

Foot-related workouts benefit the population and help prevent issues related to the diabetes mellitus (DM) and diabetic foot pain (DPN). Research utilizing worldwide exercise regimens has demonstrated benefits in musculoskeletal health, increased gait velocity, and joint range of motion. However, not all of the positive impacts last after the session, which emphasizes the significance of ongoing autonomous care and self-management. A print-based resource in the form of a suggested booklet offers patients with DPN organized and visually guided instructions on how to incorporate foot-ankle exercises into their self-management routine. The booklet has the potential to be a potent self-management tool for both public and commercial healthcare systems if the theories that it enhances clinical elements of DPN and causes advantageous biomechanical changes during stride are accurate [44].

5.6.2 LegSysTM

To gather and analyze joint kinematic data for balance evaluation and training, the study made use of verified body-worn sensor technology (LegSysTM). The sensors were affixed to various body parts, such as the lower back, thigh, and shank. The purpose of balance training activities was to provide participants with improved lower limb coordination and control over the movement of their center of mass (CoM). The training comprised a virtual obstacle-crossing activity with suitable audio-video feedback and a point-to-point ankle-reaching challenge [45].

Another body-worn sensor **(PAMSysTM)** is implanted in the T-shirt. The sensor recorded the number of steps taken when walking, standing, and sitting. For 48 hours, the sensor was inserted into a specially constructed T-shirt [45].

5.6.3 Whole-Body Vibration Exercise Training

Chronic pain is one of the main hallmarks of peripheral neuropathy caused by diabetes (DPN), which is put on by long-term hyperglycemia degrading afferent nociceptors. Balance and movement are reduced as a result of the hyperexcitation of central nerves and the resulting spontaneous nerve impulse production brought on by this injury. With WBVT, users exercise on a vibrating platform that quickly varies the length of the muscle-tendon complex, causing the muscle to contract reflexively and repeatedly, increasing the level of muscular fitness has been demonstrated that WBVT has positive benefits on blood pressure, body composition, oxygen absorption, flexibility, and muscular function. Nevertheless, there is little data on vibration therapy's effectiveness for DPN patients. Prolonged exposure to high-frequency WBV can have detrimental side effects, including accelerated degeneration of the lumbar spine, lower back discomfort, exhaustion of the muscles, and involvement in the pathophysiology of illnesses affecting the female reproductive system [46–48].

5.7 Exercise Training Recommendations by Ada (American Diabetes Association)

The exercise prescription is built on the FIIT pro approach, where F is for frequency, i.e., how frequently in a week and I represent for Intensity, i.e., how hard or how much, it might be mild, moderate, or vigorous, T stands for time, i.e., the period of exercise, and another T stands for type, which refers to the type of activity. Finally, pro stands for progression (Fig. 5.6).

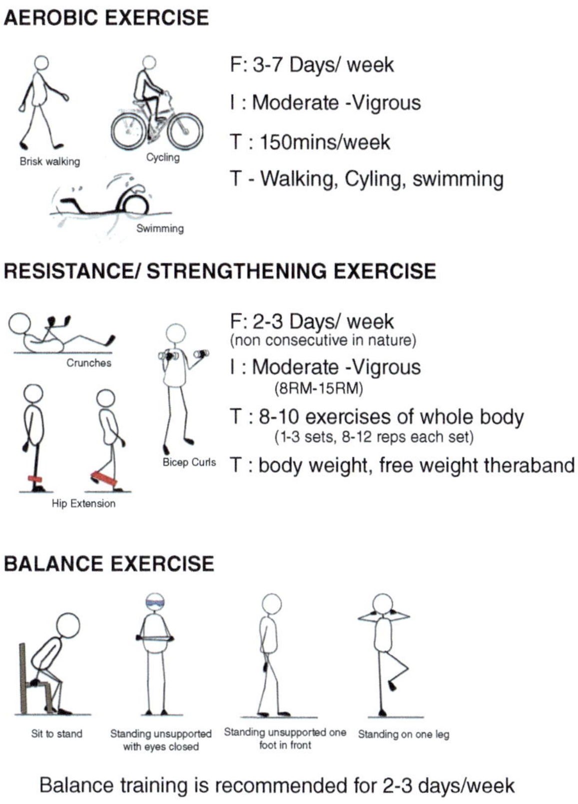

Fig. 5.6 Exercise training recommendations by American Diabetes Association (ADA). (Source: Colberg SR. Key points from the updated guidelines on exercise and diabetes. Front Endocrinol 2017;8:33. https://doi.org/10.3389/fendo.2017.00033)

It is best for adults with type 2 diabetes to exercise for at least 30 minutes each day. The amount of time spent exercising at a moderate level should be gradually increased to 150 minutes per week. Shorter bursts of hard exercise may be beneficial for people who can run at least 25 min at a pace of 6 miles per hour. If retaining fitness is the primary goal of exercise and obstacles do not prevent it, then greater emphasis should be placed on vigorous-intensity aerobic activity. For most diabetics, both HIIT and continuous fitness training are appropriate. Most adults, including those with type 2 diabetes, should engage in moderate exercise [49, 50].

Resistance exercise, at any level, should be performed two to three times a week on non-consecutive days to improve strength, balance, and everyday living skills. Start off with a moderate level of intensity and 10–15 repetitions per set. Once you consistently surpass the desired number of repetitions, you can increase the weight or resistance with fewer reps [8–10]. A higher number of sets and, finally, a higher training frequency can come after increasing resistance [51, 52].

To maintain joint range of motion, flexibility exercises for key muscle-tendon groups should be performed twice a week or more [53].

Adults with diabetes (50 years of age and older) should engage in two to three times a week exercises to maintain or enhance their balance, particularly if they have peripheral neuropathy. Yoga and tai chi can be added to enhance flexibility, strength, and balance, depending on personal preferences. Activities that strengthen the core and lower body can also be added. Maintain your focus on your flexibility and balance exercise while progressively increasing its frequency and/or duration to see progress [54].

Increasing unstructured physical activity can help manage weight and improve daily energy expenditure. Examples of such activities include cleaning the house, walking the dog, running errands, and gardening. A brief period of inactivity can enhance glycemic management, especially after meals, and lower postprandial hyperglycemia in people with prediabetes, type 1 and type 2 diabetes. Unstructured or daily activities can act as stepping stones for people with sedentary lives [55].

Maintaining better blood glucose control can benefit individuals who exercise according to the ACSM/ADA guidelines.

Like foot care and diet, exercise recommendations have to be a standard component of diabetic patients' visits to the doctor's office. A follow-up appointment should be scheduled to talk about exercise progress, obstacles, and adherence, just like with any medical advice. Using the "SMART" target mnemonic (specific, measurable, achievable, realistic, and time-oriented), adjust the workout prescription as necessary [56].

People with diabetes often engage in more physical activity and exercise, especially those who are at risk of developing diabetic peripheral neuropathy [57].

Studies indicated that persons with diabetes experienced less discomfort during and after exercise after just one session of isometric exercise. Between the pre-intervention and post-intervention periods, participants who finished at least 75% of the sessions reported significantly lower levels of pain and neuropathic symptoms. Adults with painful peripheral neuropathy who participated in a 16-week aerobic exercise program reported feeling less that their pain interfered with their lives, but their pain level remained the same [58].

One prevalent factor that encourages physical exercise in persons with diabetes is self-efficacy. The relationship between increased physical activity and self-efficacy for physical exercise is supported by cross-sectional research. Increased self-care activities for persons with diabetes were linked to higher levels of social support, which may help protect them from psychological discomfort [59, 60].

5.8 Challenges and Barriers to Exercise

5.8.1 Depression

Diabetes patients have higher rates of depression and depressed symptoms than the general population. The risk of depression in individuals with diabetes is double that of adults without the disease. Compared to males with diabetes, women with diabetes are 2–3 times more likely to experience depression. Adults with diabetes who suffer from depression find it difficult to start and maintain an exercise regimen because depression can directly erode the desire for exercise as well as other behaviors and methods that support it [61].

Over time, depression has also been connected to more severe diabetes consequences, such as mortality, myocardial infarction, stroke, amputations, blindness, and end-stage renal disease. There is a correlation between the likelihood of developing a diabetic foot ulcer (DFU) and depressed symptoms, according to recent prospective research.

5.8.2 *Anhedonia*

Poor energy and hypersomnia are examples of depressive symptoms that might interfere with exercise and exacerbate the usual obstacles to exercise that persons with diabetes describe [62].

5.8.3 *Pain*

Adults with diabetes frequently experience pain, with musculoskeletal discomfort being 1.7–2.1 times more common than in non-diabetics. Patients with diabetic neuropathy who consistently experience neuropathic pain—which is stronger in the evenings—also have sadness linked to it. It could be challenging to start exercising in this demographic because of this link [63, 64]. Still, preliminary data points to exercise as a potential pain reliever.

5.9 Conclusion

In a community that cultivates a therapeutic nurse-patient connection, holistic nursing care integrates the patient's mind, body, and spirit, leading to wholeness, harmony, and healing. To provide tailored care and treat the patient as a whole rather than in bits and parts, the holistic approach to medicine is patient-led and patient-focused. Contemporary science has been among the greatest in demonstrating the significance of soul and spirit to health, along with nursing and medicine. Not only will our patients benefit from these advancements, but healthcare workers will as well. Patients with diabetes mellitus are managed using a holistic care strategy that incorporates technology, culture, yoga, herbal food and medicine, health education, lifestyle modifications, and psychosocial and psychological support.

References

1. Khdour MR. Treatment of diabetic peripheral neuropathy: a review. J Pharm Pharmacol. 2020;72(7):863–72.
2. Zeng L, Alongkronrusmee D, van Rijn RM. An integrated perspective on diabetic, alcoholic, and drug-induced neuropathy, etiology, and treatment in the US. J Pain Res. 2017;10:219–28.
3. Bodman MA, Varacallo M. Peripheral diabetic neuropathy. Treasure Island (FL): Stat Pearls—NCBI Bookshelf; 2024. https://www.ncbi.nlm.nih.gov/books/NBK442009/.
4. Nkonge KM, Nkonge DK, Nkonge TN. Screening for diabetic peripheral neuropathy in resource-limited settings. Diabetol Metab Syndr. 2023;15(1):55.
5. Yang Y, Hu X, Zhang Q, Zou R. Diabetes mellitus and risk of falls in older adults: a systematic review and meta-analysis. Age Ageing. 2016;45(6):761–7.
6. Yang Z, Scott CA, Mao C, Tang J, Farmer AJ. Resistance exercise versus aerobic exercise for type 2 diabetes: a systematic review and meta-analysis. Sports Med. 2013;44(4):487–99.
7. Grisold A, Callaghan BC, Feldman EL. Mediators of diabetic neuropathy: is hyperglycemia the only culprit? Curr Opin Endocrinol Diabetes Obes. 2017;24(2):103–11.
8. Jørgensen IEH, Devantier L, Tankisi H, Andersen H, Khan KS. The impact of vestibular dysfunction on falls and postural instability in individuals with type 2 diabetes with and without diabetic polyneuropathy. PeerJ. 2023;11:e16382.
9. El-Refay BH, Ali OI. Efficacy of exercise rehabilitation program in improving gait of diabetic neuropathy patients. Med. J. Cairo Univ. 2014;82:225–32. Europe PMC.
10. Kanchanasamut W, Pensri P. Effects of weight-bearing exercise on a mini-trampoline on foot mobility, plantar pressure and sensation of diabetic neuropathic feet; a preliminary study. Diabet Foot Ankle. 2017;8(1):1287239.
11. Sharma J, Ahmad I, Singh AKC. Effects of exercises and manual therapy on nerve conduction studies of lower limb in patients with diabetes and diabetic peripheral neuropathy: a systematic review. Int J Diabetes Dev Ctries. 2024;44(2):241–64.
12. Colberg SR, Sigal RJ, Yardley JE, Riddell MC, Dunstan DW, Dempsey PC, et al. Physical activity/exercise and diabetes: a position statement of the American Diabetes Association. Diabetes Care. 2016;39(11):2065–79.
13. Blair SN. Changes in physical fitness and all-cause mortality. JAMA. 1995;273(14):1093–8.
14. Kim C, Choi HE, Jung H, Kang SH, Kim JH, Byun YS. Impact of aerobic exercise training on endothelial function in acute coronary syndrome. Ann Rehabil Med. 2014;38(3):388–95.
15. De Sá CA, Grudka Heizen P, Corralo VS, Gonzaga dos Santos GA, Moura Soares NM. Chronic effect of aerobic exercise on anthropometric, biochemical and hemodynamic variables in individuals with type 2 diabetes mellitus: a systematic review. Rev Andal Med Deporte. 2016;9(4):173–9.
16. Kluding PM, Pasnoor M, Singh R, D'Silva LJ, Yoo M, Billinger SA, et al. Safety of aerobic exercise in people with diabetic peripheral neuropathy: single-group clinical trial. Phys Ther. 2015;95(2):223–34.
17. Weng X, Liao S, Wang F, Wang H, Yang L. Evaluation of mindfulness training combined with aerobic exercise on neurological function and quality of life in patients with peripheral neuropathy type 2 diabetes mellitus. Contrast Media Mol Imaging. 2022;2022:7665483.
18. Kikkawa Y, Kuwabara S, Misawa S, Tamura N, Kitano Y, Ogawara K, et al. The acute effects of glycemic control on nerve conduction in human diabetics. Clin Neurophysiol. 2005;116(2):270–4.
19. Dixit S, Maiya AG, Shastry BA. Effect of aerobic exercise on peripheral nerve functions of population with diabetic peripheral neuropathy in type 2 diabetes: a single blind, parallel group randomized controlled trial. J Diabetes Complicat. 2014;28(3):332–9.
20. Azizi S, Najafi S, Rezasoltani Z, Sanati E, Zamani N, Dadarkhah A. Effects of aerobic exercise on electrophysiological features of diabetic peripheral neuropathy. Top Geriatr Rehabil. 2019;35:164–9.
21. Hamed NS, Raoof NALA. Effect of high intensity interval training on diabetic obese women with polyneuropathy: a randomized controlled clinical trial. Phys Ther Rehabil. 2014;1:4.

22. Herder C, Roden M, Ziegler D. Novel insights into sensorimotor and cardiovascular autonomic neuropathy from recent-onset diabetes and population-based cohorts. Trends Endocrinol Metab. 2019;30(4):286–98.
23. Morrison S, Colberg SR, Parson HK, Vinik AI. Exercise improves gait, reaction time and postural stability in older adults with type 2 diabetes and neuropathy. J Diabetes Complicat. 2014;28(5):715–22.
24. Gohel MG, Chacko AN. Serum GGT activity and hsCRP level in patients with type 2 diabetes mellitus with good and poor glycemic control: an evidence linking oxidative stress, inflammation and glycemic control. J Diabetes Metab Disord. 2013;12(1):56.
25. Stone MH, Stone M, Sands WA. Principles and practice of resistance training. Champaign, IL: Human Kinetics; 2007.
26. Faigenbaum AD, Kraemer WJ, Blimkie CJR, Jeffreys I, Micheli LJ, Nitka M, et al. Youth resistance training: updated position statement paper from the National Strength and Conditioning Association. J Strength Cond Res. 2009;23(Suppl 5):S60–79.
27. Iglay HB, Thyfault JP, Apolzan JW, Campbell WW. Resistance training and dietary protein: effects on glucose tolerance and contents of skeletal muscle insulin signaling proteins in older persons. Am J Clin Nutr. 2007;85(4):1005–13.
28. Cook MD, Heffernan KS, Ranadive S, Woods JA, Fernhall B. Effect of resistance training on biomarkers of vascular function and oxidative stress in young African-American and Caucasian men. J Hum Hypertens. 2013;27(6):388–92.
29. Tilling LM, Darawil K, Britton M. Falls as a complication of diabetes mellitus in older people. J Diabetes Complicat. 2006;20(3):158–62.
30. Handsaker JC, Brown SJ, Bowling FL, Cooper G, Maganaris CN, Boulton AJM, et al. Contributory factors to unsteadiness during walking up and down stairs in patients with diabetic peripheral neuropathy. Diabetes Care. 2014;37(11):3047–53.
31. Handsaker JC, Brown SJ, Bowling FL, Maganaris CN, Boulton AJM, Reeves ND. Resistance exercise training increases lower limb speed of strength generation during stair ascent and descent in people with diabetic peripheral neuropathy. Diabet Med. 2015;33(1):97–104.
32. Saleki M, Nadi M, Marandi S, Esfarjani F, Mohammadi M. The comparison between effects of 12 weeks combined training and vitamin D supplement on improvement of sensory-motor neuropathy in type 2 diabetic women. Adv Biomed Res. 2017;6(1):55.
33. Song CH, Petrofsky JS, Lee SW, Lee KJ, Yim JE. Effects of an exercise program on balance and trunk proprioception in older adults with diabetic neuropathies. Diabetes Technol Ther. 2011;13(8):803–11.
34. Willis Boslego LA, Munterfering Phillips CE, Atler KE, Tracy BL, Van Puymbroeck M, Schmid AA. Impact of yoga on balance, balance confidence and occupational performance for adults with diabetic peripheral neuropathy: a pilot study. Br J Occup Ther. 2017;80(3):155–62.
35. Kanjirathingal J, Mullerpatan R, Nehete G, Raghuram N. Effect of yogasana intervention on standing balance performance among people with diabetic peripheral neuropathy: a pilot study. Int J Yoga. 2021;14(1):60–70.
36. Kelley K, Slattery K, Apollo K. An electromyographic analysis of selected asana in experienced yogic practitioners. J Bodyw Mov Ther. 2018;22(1):152–8.
37. Wang MY, Yu SS, Hashish R, Samarawickrame SD, Kazadi L, Greendale GA, Salem G. The biomechanical demands of standing yoga pose in seniors: the Yoga empowers seniors' study (YESS). BMC Complement Altern Med. 2013;13:8.
38. Ahn S, Song R. Effects of Tai Chi Exercise on glucose control, neuropathy scores, balance, and quality of life in patients with type 2 diabetes and neuropathy. J Altern Complement Med. 2012;18(12):1172–8.
39. Jagga V, Suman R. Wobble board-based exercises and Swiss ball-based exercises in improving balance and mobility in patients with diabetic neuropathy. Korean J Physiol Pharmacol. 2024;28(1):318–22.

40. Hung ES-W, Chen S-C, Chang F-C, Shiao Y, Peng C-W, Lai C-H. Effects of interactive video game-based exercise on balance in diabetic patients with peripheral neuropathy: an open-level, Crossover Pilot Study. Evid Based Complement Alternat Med. 2019;2019:4540709.
41. Shabbott BA, Sainburg RL. Learning a visuomotor rotation: simultaneous visual and proprioceptive information is crucial for visuomotor remapping. Exp Brain Res. 2010;203(1):75–87.
42. Prókai J, Murlasits Z, Bánhidi M, Csóka L, Gréci V, Atlasz T, et al. The effects of a 12-week-long sand exercise training program on neuromechanical and functional parameters in type II diabetic patients with neuropathy. Int J Environ Res Public Health. 2023;20(7):5413.
43. Ansari A, Karimizadeh Ardakani M, Akoochakian M. Effects of weight-bearing exercise on a mini-trampoline, and foot-ankle therapeutic exercise program on foot-ankle functionality in people with diabetic peripheral neuropathy. Phys Treatments—Spec Phys Ther J. 2022;12(4):291–302.
44. Silva EQ, Suda EY, Santos DP, et al. Effect of an educational booklet for prevention and treatment of foot musculoskeletal dysfunctions in people with diabetic neuropathy: the FOotCAre (FOCA) trial II, a study protocol of a randomized controlled trial. Trials. 2020;21(1):180.
45. Mansfield A, Wong JS, Bryce J, Knorr S, Patterson KK, Inness EL. Objective fall risk detection in stroke survivors using wearable sensor technology: a feasibility study. Top Stroke Rehabil. 2016;23(6):422–30.
46. Machado A, García-López D, González-Gallego J, Garatachea N. Whole-body vibration training increases muscle strength and mass in older women: a randomized controlled trial. Scand J Med Sci Sports. 2009;20(2):200–7.
47. Abercromby AFJ, Amonette WE, Layne CS, McFarlin BK, Hinman MR, Paloski WH. Vibration exposure and biodynamic responses during whole-body vibration training. Med Sci Sports Exerc. 2007;39(10):1794–800.
48. Camacho-Cardenosa M, Camacho-Cardenosa A, Burtscher M, Brazo-Sayavera J, Tomas-Carus P, Olcina G, et al. Effects of whole-body vibration training combined with cyclic hypoxia on bone mineral density in elderly people. Front Physiol. 2019;10:1122.
49. Jelleyman C, Yates T, O'Donovan G, Gray LJ, King JA, Khunti K, et al. The effects of high-intensity interval training on glucose regulation and insulin resistance: a meta-analysis. Obes Rev. 2015;16(11):942–61.
50. Tonoli C, Heyman E, Roelands B, Buyse L, Cheung SS, Berthoin S, et al. Effects of different Types of acute and chronic (training) exercise on glycaemic control in type 1 diabetes mellitus. Sports Med. 2012;42(12):1059–80.
51. King AC, Powell KE, Kraus WE. The US Physical Activity Guidelines Advisory Committee Report—introduction. Med Sci Sports Exerc. 2019;51(6):1203–5.
52. Willey KA, Singh MAF. Battling insulin resistance in elderly obese people with type 2 diabetes. Diabetes Care. 2003;26(5):1580–8.
53. Garber CE, Blissmer B, Deschenes MR, Franklin BA, Lamonte MJ, Lee I-M, et al. Quantity and quality of exercise for developing and maintaining cardiorespiratory, musculoskeletal, and neuromotor fitness in apparently healthy adults. Med Sci Sports Exerc. 2011;43(7):1334–59.
54. Morrison S, Colberg SR, Mariano M, Parson HK, Vinik AI. Balance training reduces falls risk in older individuals with type 2 diabetes. Diabetes Care. 2010;33(4):748–50.
55. Umpierre D, Ribeiro PA, Kramer CK, Leitão CB, Zucatti AT, Azevedo MJ, Gross JL, Ribeiro JP, Schaan BD. Physical activity advice only or structured exercise training and association with HbA1c levels in type 2 diabetes: a systematic review and meta-analysis. JAMA. 2011;305(17):1790–9.
56. Dugan JA. Exercise recommendations for patients with type 2 diabetes. J Am Acad Phys Assist. 2016;29(10):13–8.
57. LeMaster JW, Mueller MJ, Reiber GE, Mehr DR, Madsen RW, Conn VS. Effect of weight-bearing activity on foot ulcer incidence in people with diabetic peripheral neuropathy: feet first randomized controlled trial. Phys Ther. 2008;88(11):1385–98.
58. Knauf MT, Koltyn KF. Exercise-induced modulation of pain in adults with and without painful diabetic neuropathy. J Pain. 2014;15(6):656–63.

59. Walker RJ, Gebregziabher M, Martin-Harris B, Egede LE. Understanding the influence of psychological and socioeconomic factors on diabetes self-care using structured equation modeling. Patient Educ Couns. 2015;98(1):34–40.
60. Tulloch H, Sweet SN, Fortier M, Capstick G, Kenny GP, Sigal RJ. Exercise facilitators and barriers from adoption to maintenance in the diabetes aerobic and resistance exercise trial. Can J Diabetes. 2013;37(6):367–74.
61. Crews RT, Schneider KL, Yalla SV, Reeves ND, Vileikyte L. Physiological and psychological challenges of increasing physical activity and exercise in patients at risk of diabetic foot ulcers: a critical review. Diabetes Metab Res Rev. 2016;32(8):791–804.
62. Vickers KS, Nies MA, Patten CA, Dierkhising R, Smith SA. Patients with diabetes and depression may need additional support for exercise. Am J Health Behav. 2006;30(4):353–62.
63. Barrett AM, Lucero MA, Le T, Robinson RL, Dworkin RH, Chappell AS. Epidemiology, public health burden, and treatment of diabetic peripheral neuropathic pain: a review. Pain Med. 2007;8(2):S50–62.
64. daCosta DiBonaventura M, Cappelleri JC, Joshi AV. A longitudinal assessment of painful diabetic peripheral neuropathy on health status, productivity, and health care utilization and cost. Pain Med. 2011;12(1):118–26.

Chapter 6
Electrotherapy Interventions for Diabetic Peripheral Neuropathy

Kirti Chhabra and Neha Kashyap

Contents

6.1 Introduction

In the world, diabetic peripheral neuropathy, or DPN, is thought to be the commonest type of neuropathy. About 75% of all peripheral neuropathies are symmetrical peripheral polyneuropathy. It is marked by pain, ulcers on the legs, and the possibility of lower limb amputation. To be more precise, 50% of individuals with DPN experience foot ulcers at least once in their lives. Pain and loss of feeling are symptoms that might cause falls, related injuries like sprains, limits on everyday activities, despair, and ultimately a lower quality of life [1].

K. Chhabra (✉) · N. Kashyap
MM Institute of Physiotherapy & Rehabilitation, Maharishi Markandeshwar (Deemed to be University), Ambala, Haryana, India
e-mail: neha.kashyup@mmumullana.org

© The Author(s), under exclusive license to Springer Nature Singapore Pte Ltd. 2024

M. Goyal, K. Goyal (eds.), *Rehabilitation in Diabetic Peripheral Neuropathy*,
https://doi.org/10.1007/978-981-97-9290-0_6

An interdisciplinary approach to managing diabetic peripheral neuropathy (DPN) is necessary.

This approach should focus on managing vascular risk factors, changing lifestyle behavior with food and exercise [2], maintaining appropriate foot hygiene, and managing pain. For health scientists, treating neuropathic pain is quite challenging because it is frequently persistent and linked to low patient satisfaction with therapy [3]. Although many individuals may not respond well to medication and may also encounter side effects that worsen their overall condition, medication can assist manage pain. Therefore, other treatment approaches are being explored for the management of diabetic neuropathic pain [4].

Electrotherapy is one approach that has been demonstrated to improve endoneurial blood flow and microcirculation. Given that diabetic peripheral neuropathy patients have reduced microcirculation in their peripheral nerves, electrotherapy may be beneficial. It's also noteworthy that electrotherapy has a metabolic influence on the muscle's ability to oxidize more fuel. Electrical stimulation has also an impact on the morphological and metabolic characteristics of paralyzed muscles [5].

Electrotherapy techniques include transcranial direct current stimulation (tDCS), repetitive transcranial magnetic stimulation (rTMS), transcutaneous electrical nerve stimulation (TENS), low-level laser therapy (LLLT), electromagnetic fields, plantar electrical stimulation (PES), percutaneous electrical nerve stimulation (PENS), found to be effective in patients with diabetic peripheral neuropathy (DPN).

6.2 Different Interventions for DPN

6.2.1 TENS: Types and Properties

TENS is a non-invasive, analgesic method utilized for an array of neuropathic concerns [6].

TENS can be classified into three types: (Table 6.1)

(a) Intense TENS (high intensity and high frequency). This is because different stimulus parameters for TENS may activate different populations of nerve fibers [7].
(b) Acupuncture-like TENS (high intensity and low frequency), and
(c) Conventional TENS with varying intensity and frequency (both low intensity and high frequency)

Table 6.1 below provides specific information on the attributes for different TENS categories [7]

Table 6.1 Transcutaneous electrical nerve stimulation types and treatment parameters

Types	Stimulation	Intensity/Frequency	Electrode placement (Fig. 6.1)
Conventional TENS	Large diameter, Aβ fibers	Below the point of threshold for pain, high frequency (> 10 Hz)	Placed around painful region
Acupuncture-like TENS	Small diameter, A δ & C fibers	Surpassing the threshold for tolerance to pain, low frequency (2–4 Hz)	Electrodes are situated far away from the apprehensive region
Intense TENS	Small diameter, A δ fibers	Attaining the threshold for pain tolerance, high frequency (>200 Hz)	Electrodes are placed on or near the painful area

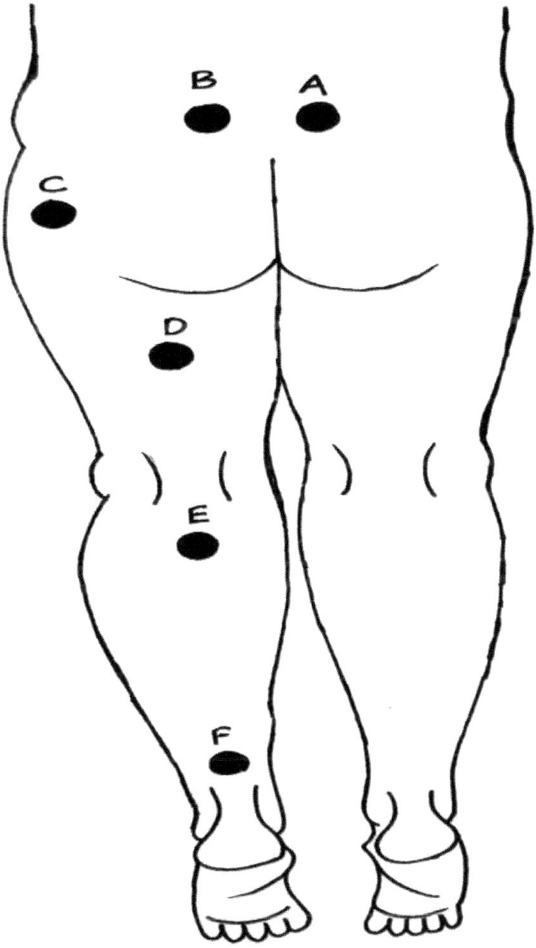

Fig. 6.1 Electrode placement of TENS dermatomal for diabetic peripheral neuropathy. A: L4-L5 Region. B: L4-L5 Region. C: Belly of Piriformis muscle. D: Mid-thigh. E: Distal to Popliteal Fossa. F: Achilles Tendon

6.2.1.1 Neurobiological Mechanisms

Analgesic effects produced by TENS are brought by a variety of neurobiological mechanisms that affect the central and peripheral nerve systems. Specifically, administering electrical pulses to the skin's surface may activate nerve fibers, which may modify electrical transmission, widen blood vessels, and release endogenous opioids, all of which may reduce neuropathic pain [8, 9].

There are three distinct analgesic processes associated with different forms of TENS: peripheral, segmental, and extra segmental [7]. Because conventional TENS can lead to suppression at particular segments in nociceptive spinal transmission route at the dorsal horn, it is thought to primarily be associated with segmental mechanisms. Since descending pain inhibition system can be recruited to induce analgesia, extra segmental mechanisms are thought to be substantially responsible for the effects of TENS and strong TENS both strong and ordinary TENS, which are both given at a high frequency, have also been linked to peripheral processes because they can elicit peripheral blockage of afferent impulses [7].

6.2.1.1.1 Peripheral Mechanisms

TENS therapy can stimulate nerve impulses to travel along the nerve axon away from the central nervous system. This is known as antidromic activation, and it can occur in peripheral afferent nerves with both standard and severe TENS. As antidromic nerve impulses collide with and also inhibit afferent impulses emanating via damaged tissue, the antidromic activation might lead to the peripheral blocking of nociceptive impulses [10, 11].

Conventional TENS-induced peripheral blockage generally occurs in fibers of big diameter (e.g., Aβ fibers), which may result in a "busy line effect" that helps some people with allodynia feel better. It is more noticeable to see peripheral nociceptive impulse blocking with the severe TENS treatment. Intense TENS would cause nerve impulses in Aδ fibers to interfere with nociceptive impulses coming from the damaged tissue. In isolated nerves, TENS can lower the amplitude and conduction velocity of Aβ and Aδ fiber action potentials [7].

6.2.1.1.2 Central Mechanisms

The primary mechanism of action of conventional TENS is in the segmental processes, whereby electrical stimulation of large-diameter Aβ fibers can activate the dorsal horn of the spinal cord's inhibitory neurons, thereby decreasing the rate at which projection neurons fire [7]. Gate control theory of pain given by Melzack and Wall's is consistent with the segmental processes [12]. Non-nociceptive inputs "close the gates" on nerves to nociceptive signals, preventing nociceptive impulses from entering the central nervous system [7].

By activating the descending pain inhibition system, TENS that resembles acupuncture and intense TENS can have analgesic benefits [13]. The phenomenon known as diffuse noxious inhibitory control (DNIC) is more closely linked to their analgesic effects. DNIC is the result of diffuse descending inhibition of nociception (DNIC) caused by endogenous opioid releases in the rostral ventral medulla (RVM) and periaqueductal gray (PAG) in response to a severe noxious input [14, 15]. In addition to recruiting the PAG-RVM network, analgesic benefits can also be attained by stimulating neurons in the medullary subnucleus reticularis dorsalis, a member of the DNIC system. Additionally, additional segmental processes could be involved in the classic TENS's analgesic effects [16].

Hence, TENS is considered as an effective and safe treatment in DPNP and it is advised to use TENS to DPNP sufferers as a non-pharmacological method of pain management [7].

6.2.2 *Low-Power Laser Therapy (LLLT)*

LLLT, or low-laser therapy, is a different term for soft laser. It makes use of a low-power laser to induce a biological reaction at wavelengths between 632 and 1064 nm. (1–1000 mW) [17, 18].

Low-level lasers can be either of the following:

(a) Helium-Neon laser (He-Ne), which emits red light at 632.8 nm
(b) Aluminum Gallium Arsenide (Al Ga As) or laser diode, which emits infrared light at 780–830 nm.
(c) A combination of Helium-Neon diode and laser [19].

There is no noise, vibration, or heat generated during this non-invasive procedure [17, 18]. Red and near-infrared light at low level is emitted onto the skin or tissue. It is referred to as a low-level laser since it uses far less light than other types of laser therapy [20].

Additionally, by increasing the synthesis of collagen and reducing oxidative stress as well as increasing oxygen consumption by quickening the tempo of the redox reaction, promoting the production of ATP (adenosine triphosphate) and anti-inflammatory cytokines, LLLT may be able to lessen pain [21].

In addition to inducing collagen and protein production, LLLT also relieves pain, repairs damaged nerve fibers more quickly, and causes tissue repair. It is also utilized to promote nerve regeneration and to alleviate inflammation and tissue hypoxia/ischemia in nerve entrapment neuropathy [22].

6.2.2.1 Mechanism of Action: LLLT in DPN

LLLT induces a photochemical reaction in the cell that is referred to as photo bio-modulation or bio-stimulation. Thermal processes and photonic radiation are responsible for the biological response that was attained. This can be accomplished by having the mitochondrial chromophore, cytochrome oxidase, absorb red light, which sets off a chain of events in the mitochondria that have a bio-stimulation impact [21].

The primary pathophysiological cause leading to the development of diabetic neuropathy is hyper glycemia. It sets off several processes that result in diabetic neuropathy, including the production of free radicals, the activation of the polyol pathway, the erroneous regulation of neurotrophic factors, and the production of glycation end products. Diabetes ulcers, which are thought to be the main source of morbidity in diabetes patients, are the consequence of a series of events set off by neuronal dysfunction that results in loss of pain perception [22].

LLLT hastens the process of healing of tissue that is injured and photo acceptor molecules undergo electronic excitation as a result of the effects of laser light, which starts at the cellular and subcellular levels. This is accomplished by connecting with the carboxyl-terminal binding protein (CtBP), a corepressor that is involved in transcriptional pathways critical to the control of the cell cycle. The electrical excitation of photo acceptors was proposed to trigger four probable events: alterations in single- and superoxide production, redox control by NAD+ and NADH, and changes in metabolic activity [22].

Electron transport in the mitochondrial membrane promotes cell metabolism and proliferation, including the production of ATP from ADP, which may show up as increased protein synthesis and DNA synthesis. This helps wounded nerve cells repair more quickly and reduces pain perception [22].

Additionally, LLLT reduces inflammation by activating microcirculation, altering prostaglandin levels, restoring normal osmotic pressure, and removing edema. Following this anti-inflammatory impact, pain is subsequently managed. Moreover, the reflexogenic impact of LLLT is linked to the activation of physiological function by first irritating nerve endings and then excitation of nerve centers [23].

Diabetes has been shown to be linked to oxidative stress as a result of protein glycosylation and autoxidation of glucose (Al-Faris, 2010). Oxidative and nitrosative stress, which can result in endothelial dysfunction, insulin resistance, and changes in the quantity and functions of pancreatic ς cells, is brought on by a persistent rise in reactive oxygen species and reactive nitrogen species concurrent with a decrease in antioxidant activity. Hence, LLLT's anti-inflammatory properties may be responsible for the therapeutic benefit of lowering this oxidative stress [21].

When comparing patients with DPN to placebo, those who got photon stimulation over time had a significant improvement in sensation and a drop in pain scores.

Distressingly, diabetes mellitus can have DPN, which increases morbidity and death significantly. These individuals now have much lower quality of life due to a lack of a viable therapeutic option. LLLT is now becoming more and more of a viable treatment option in patients with DPN [21].

Table 6.2 Low-level laser therapy as intervention in DPN [21]

Neuropathy type	Laser parameters [laser power (nm), energy density (J/cm^2)	Intervention duration	Outcome
Diabetic peripheral neuropathy	The wavelength used mostly between 800 and 900 nm and energy density being used frequently- (3–4 J/cm^2)	Usually given for a time frame of 10 days to 4 weeks.	On using VAS, NCS and TCSS as an outcome measure, results are effective with LLLT usage.
Diabetic sensorimotor polyneuropathy			
Distal symmetric neuropathy			

It was evident that LLLT is a safe, economical, non-invasive, and effective way to treat DPN. Pain relief was one of LLLT's primary outcomes. Treatment factors and radiation levels affected the outcome [21]. (Table 6.2).

Therefore, it is concluded that LLLT is an effective treatment modality in relieving pain, redistributing plantar pressure and improving NCV in patients with DPN [21].

6.2.3 Transcranial Direct Current Stimulation (TDCS)

Neuromodulation uses a variety of stimulation techniques to correct or balance out various imbalances in the central, peripheral, or autonomic nervous systems [24] and one of the new non-invasive techniques called TDCS is used with the objective to treat neuropathic pain caused by PNP. Anodal or cathodal stimulation, which depolarizes (activates; anodal tDCS) and hyperpolarizes (inhibits; cathodal tDCS) cortical circuits, is the purpose of TDCS, a low-amplitude electrical current administered to the cortex using scalp electrodes [25].

6.2.3.1 Treatment Procedure: TDCS

6.2.3.1.1 Application Procedure

- Positioning of the anode electrode is above the main motor cortex (m1) and positioning of the cathode electrode is above the supra-orbital region. The DC was started out increasing in a ramp-like style and continued for a long time till reaching 1–2 mA (Fig. 6.2).
- If the individual has any of the following symptoms: headache, extreme itching or numbness under the electrode locations, dizziness, or vomiting, the session would be ended.

  Treatment duration: 20 min with 1–2 mA of intensity, five consecutive days [26].

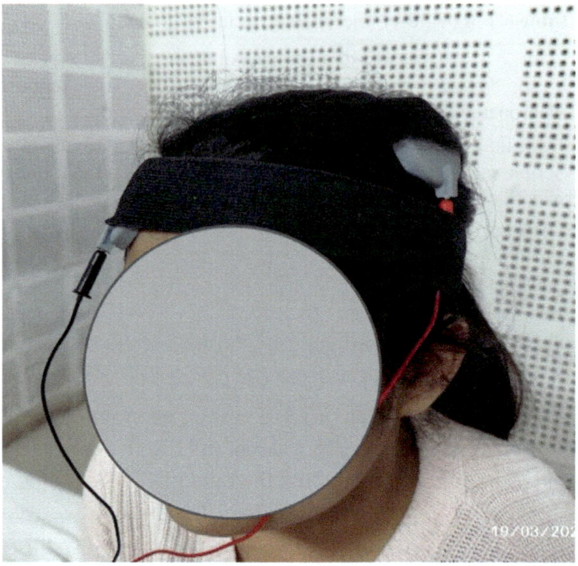

Fig. 6.2 Electrode placement of tDCS according to 10:20 EEG electrode placement system for DPN patients

6.2.3.2 Mechanism of Function: TDCS

The polarity-based changes in the resting membrane potential of the neurons under the electrodes, which transforms neuronal excitation at the stimulation site and surrounding areas, have been shown to be the mechanism of action of transcutaneous direct current stimulation (tDCS). Because the anode tends to activate bigger neuronal activities, it is usually placed close to the target location, such as the first motor area (m1), vertex (c3 or c4), or frontal (f3 or f4) regions [26].

When it comes to managing NP usage of various places for stimulation, the major motor area (M1) and dorsolateral prefrontal cortex (DLPFC) are the main regions of interest for transcranial magnetic stimulation (tDCS). Primary motor cortex works alongside the somatosensory system and communicates with the brain regions linked to pain perception while dorsolateral prefrontal cortex (DLPFC) has its significance in emotional control and cognitive function. Thus, F3 stimulation may have an indirect impact on pain perception by affecting the cognitive and emotional aspects of pain. The brain's pain processing network does, in fact, involve the left DLPFC. Pain perception can be altered by tDCS of the DLPFC, which can affect how the brain interprets pain signals [27].

Diabetes mellitus (DM) has the potential to impact central nervous system functions, such as cognition, motor function, and pain perception. Changes in neurogenesis, angiogenesis, neural protection, and plasticity have resulted from the use of neuromodulation on people with vascular illnesses affecting the central nervous system. These changes have improved pain management, enhanced muscle performance, and allowed for functional recovery. There have been suggestions that DCS can be employed as an adjuvant therapy in functional rehabilitation programs [28].

As diabetic polyneuropathy worsens, somatosensory inputs are reduced, which results in a decline in muscle function and functional losses. During transcranial magnetic stimulation (tDCS) therapy, anodal stimulation may facilitate the rise in M1 activity, leading to enhancements in motor function. Neuromodulation seeks to increase excitability in the motor cortex by altering deep brain areas associated with pain control and motor function. Anodal M1 tDCS has the potential to lengthen endurance times, reduce discomfort in the muscles associated with fatigue, enhance synergist muscle coupling, and boost motivation. These advantages might affect day-to-day activities and enhance functionality, well-being, and physical fitness in patient having DPN [28].

Since tDCS significantly reduces neuropathic pain, it is a useful method for enhancing a patient's overall quality of life who has DPN. Thus, tDCS directly affects applied cognition, general concern, and depression while lowering anxiety and fatigue and enhancing upper and lower limb activities [26].

6.2.4 Repetitive Transcranial Magnetic Stimulation (rTMS)

Repeated transcranial magnetic stimulation (rTMS) is a safe, non-invasive therapy method that creates a magnetic field around the head using an electromagnetic coil. rTMS modifies trans-synaptic excitability at distant regions and cortical excitability at the stimulation site. It can be stated that repetitive transcranial magnetic stimulation (rTMS) at low frequencies (51 Hz) has been shown to have inhibitory effects, while high frequencies (= 5 Hz) have been shown to produce excitatory effects. Specifically, high-frequency stimulation (≥5 Hz) increases cortical excitability, while low-frequency stimulation (1 Hz) decreases it [29].

6.2.4.1 Application of rTMS in DPN

- Initiating high-frequency repeated transcranial magnetic stimulation (HF-rTMS) at 10 Hz could include applying an intensity ranging from 80% to 90% of the resting motor threshold (RMT) to the hands' primary motor cortex, regardless of the patient's location or source of pain.
- The main cerebral cortex of the hands on the side opposite the pain location may be stimulated in cases of oriented laterally neuropathic discomfort. Nonetheless, it has been observed that the left cerebral cortex may act as the stimulation focal site in situations of generalized neurological pain.
- It is recommended that after six or seven sessions of therapy, healthcare experts reevaluate if pain relief has increased to the point where it is a two on a numerical scale that ranges from 0 to 10 or if it surpasses 30% of the baseline evaluation. The principal cognitive cortex, which is connected to the sensations and movement abilities of one's face and limbs, could be another area of stimulation to try if the patient doesn't improve after the first course of treatment.

- In the event that no response is received, the final, although no less significant, attention should be directed to the left dorsolateral prefrontal cortex (DLPFC), stimulating at 100–110% of the resting motor threshold (RMT) utilizing the F3 localization technique. Located near the insular cortex, the additional sensory cortex is considered to have an integral part in the sense of pain [29].

The secondary somatosensory brain and its insular counterpart are shown to have significant functional connections during pain episodes. Subcortical networks and cortico-cortical links likely allow rTMS to promote both the triggering location and distant areas undergo changes. Because of this, rTMS might have analgesic effects across multiple neural network regions. After the successful first course of treatment, the dosage is progressively reduced from once in two weeks to a single session monthly [29].

6.2.4.2 Mechanism of Neuropathic Pain Reduction

rTMS has varying analgesic effects depending on several criteria. Furthermore, the fundamental mechanism of rTMS remains not widely understood. Thus, with an emphasis on neuropathic pain, we attempted to suggest potential pathways pertaining to HF- and (low frequency) LF-rTMS [29] (Fig. 6.3).

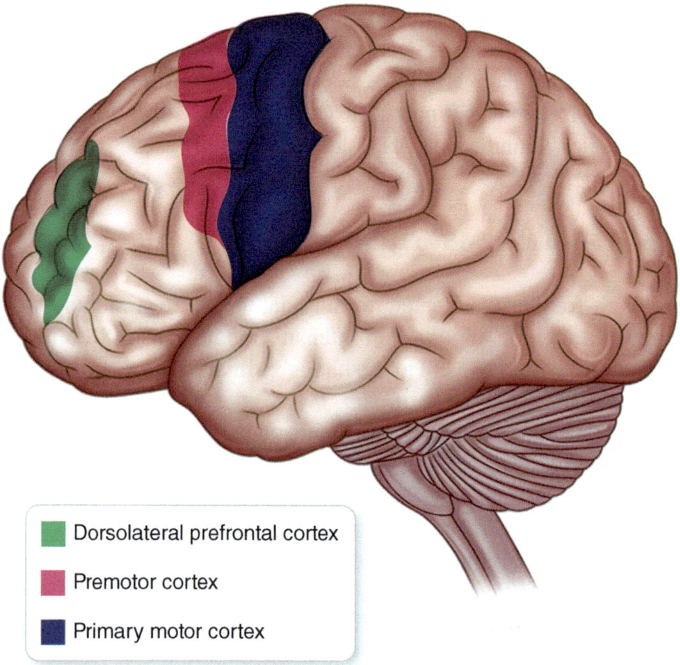

Fig. 6.3 "Diagrammatic layout showing different areas of brain involved in reducing neuropathic pain (primary motor cortex, premotor cortex and dorsolateral prefrontal cortex. (Adapted from Tsai et al. [29], licensed under CC-BY 4.0)

6.2.4.2.1 HF-rTMS

It was suggested that the analgesic effects of motor cortex stimulation and HF-rTMS of the primary motor cortex on pain and affective-emotional perception would be similar. The pathways from the caudal anterior cingulate cortex to the posterior insula, the orbitofrontal cortex to the posterior thalamus, and the periaqueductal gray to the rostroventromedial medulla are thought to be in charge of (1) raising the pain threshold, (2) regulating emotion and mood, and (3) blocking descending pain impulses. The depolarization sensitivity resulting from aberrant adaptation or impairment to pain pathways was lessened by the suggested methods.

Moreover, a technique known as neuro-navigation pinpoints specific intracranial structures by assembling a collection of neural pictures. While both HF-rTMS neuro-navigated as well as non-navigated HF-rTMS that target the primary motor area appeared to be beneficial, the last one appeared to have longer-lasting analgesic benefits in individuals with localized neuropathic pain [29].

6.2.4.2.2 LFRTMS

The prefrontal cortex's LF-rTMS found its way to enhance interleukin-10 (IL-10), tumor necrosis factor-alpha (TNF-α), and regional brain-derived neurotrophic factor (BDNF) in rats. According to current theories, BDNF functions as both a neuromediator cascade that causes prolonged synaptic stimulation and a biological indicator of activity in neurons and excitability in the cortex.

Interleukin-10 (IL-10), the alpha form of tumor necrosis factor (TNF-α), and regional neurotrophic factor from the brain (BDNF) were reported to be enhanced in rats by the prefrontal cortex's LF-rTMS. Based on current hypotheses, BDNF serves as a biological indicator of activity in neurons and excitability in the cortex, as well as a neuro-mediator cascade that produces prolonged synaptic stimulation [29].

6.2.4.3 rTMS for Neuropathic Pain Comorbidities

Individuals who experience persistent neurological discomfort frequently have coexisting diseases such as mood problems and anxiety. Major depressive disorders and depression were prevalent in 65.6% of patients with persistent neuropathic pain, respectively. It was demonstrated that depressed patients' DLPFC connection was unbalanced [29].

To address depression and enhance neuronal activity, HF-rTMS was applied to the left DLPFC. The DLPFC is associated with pain suppression and along the descending pain pathways becomes active in reaction to unpleasant stimuli. Additionally, a negative connection between pain and left DLPFC activity was discovered. According to a neurophysiological study, motor-evoked potential characteristics were changed by conditioned transcranial magnetic stimulation of the frontal cortex, indicating the presence of a cortico-cortical association [29, 30].

According to the available data, the DLPFC's HF-rTMS may have brief analgesic benefits [31]; however, in individuals with neuropathic pain, HF-rTMS of the primary motor cortex may have more substantial analgesic effects [32]. Moreover, it is clear that pain reliever advantages of neither the indirect alleviation of depression nor the mediation or indication of concomitant psychiatric diseases were linked to HF-rTMS [29].

Furthermore, among DPN patients receiving rTMS, higher scores on the SF-36 PCS and SF-36 MCS, respectively, imply a superior quality of life on the physical and mental levels [33].

rTMS can be used to treat neuropathic pain in a safe and efficient manner. Based on the existing research, neuropathic pain can be effectively treated by 10 Hz HF-rTMS of the primary motor cortex, particularly in those with diabetic neuropathy. Raising the pain threshold, blocking pain impulses, adjusting imbalanced functional connectivity in the brain cortex, it is anticipated that rTMS has analgesic properties through regulating neurotrophins as well as elevating endogenous opioids and cytokines that suppress inflammation. Additionally, the patients' physical and mental well-being improved after receiving rTMS treatment. Therefore, we believe that rTMS is a beneficial therapeutic option for those with DPN [29].

6.2.4.4 Contraindications

- As magnetic field may cause implanted equipment to unset or malfunction, intracranial metallic hardware, including electrodes, brain stimulators, epidural cortical stimulators, aneurysm clips, and ventriculoperitoneal shunts with coils, stents, and programming, is strictly contraindicated to rTMS.
- Due to insufficient safety data, individuals who have implanted electronic devices, such as pacemakers, implantable cardioverter defibrillators, spinal cord stimulators, and cochlear implants, shouldn't utilize rTMS. According to a study, rTMS seems secure for electrical devices as long as the pulse generator inside is kept apart from the rTMS coil. Furthermore, patients who have recently had electrical equipment that is suitable for magnetic resonance imaging inserted are regarded to be reasonably safe candidates for rTMS administration; nonetheless, larger-scale research is necessary to ensure long-term monitoring.
- Because of the possible hazards to the developing fetus, rTMS is usually not recommended during pregnancy. Nonetheless, the information that is now available suggests that the fetus is not negatively impacted [29].

6.2.4.5 Adverse Effects

- The majority of side effects, which range from mild to severe, include headache, nausea, tinnitus, hearing loss, headache, and soreness in the scalp. For instance, syncope and seizures are serious conditions that can occasionally happen. It has been shown that headaches represent 9.7% of adverse events, followed by scalp discomfort at 9.3% and nausea at 5%.

- Moreover, rTMS generates strong, short clicks made by coils. Maximum sound pressure for these noises is for operators, between 96 and 125 dB, and between 110 and 139 dB for receivers. These sounds are above the 85 dB threshold, which can result in temporary or permanent hearing damage. Even in those with normal hearing, the click noises produced by when stimulated, rTMS have the ability to significantly increase the auditory threshold and impede hearing. However, the auditory threshold increase did not persist for more than an hour following a single 20-minute rTMS session.
- According to research, rTMS-related seizures are incredibly rare and typically self-limited. Individuals undergoing HF-rTMS, LF-rTMS, intermittent theta burst rTMS, and continuous theta burst rTMS had an estimated likelihood of a seizure each session of 0.05%, 0.03%, 0.06%, and 0%, respectively. When rTMS was administered according to the published criteria to individuals who weren't at risk of experiencing seizures, such as those with brain tumors, severe head trauma, concussions, neurologic diseases, or those using drugs that reduce the seizure threshold, no seizures were documented. Further contraindications and precautions of rTMS are enlisted in Table 6.3.

Table 6.3 Contraindications and negative consequences of rTMS [29]

Sr no.	Contraindications	Negative consequences
1.	Metallic devices used inside the brain, including electrodes, coils, stents, brain stimulators, epidural cortical stimulators, aneurysm clips, and programmable ventriculoperitoneal shunts	1. Epilepsy (<1%)
2.	Implanted electronic devices, such as pacemakers, implantable cardioverter defibrillators, spinal cord stimulators, and cochlear implants	2. Having syncope
3.	Seizures' history, epilepsy, and seizures connected to transcranial magnetic stimulation.	3. Pain and discomfort in the scalp
4.	Syncope history	4. Dizziness
5.	History of cerebral lesion caused by vascular, traumatic, tumorous, infectious, or metabolic processes	5. Headache (most prevalent)
6.	Medications that may decrease the threshold for seizures	6. Having nausea and vomiting
7.	Pregnancy: According to the information currently available, there are no negative consequences on the fetus.	7. Loss of hearing and ringing in the ear

6.2.5 Plantar Electrical Stimulation (PES)

Using electrotherapy equipment to stimulate the plantar surface is known as plantar electrical stimulation. Plantar electrical stimulation is a safe, effective, and side-effect-free way to improve motor function in people with DPN [34].

6.2.5.1 Indications and Benefits

- After daily electrical stimulation, people with DPN are assumed to have improved plantar skin perfusion, which leads to an improvement in plantar sensation [34].
- In DPN patients, decreased local blood flow can result in substances that impede neural signals and oxidative stress.
- Electrical stimulation has been shown to have many advantages, including helping to heal wounds and increasing skin perfusion by releasing vascular endothelial growth factor.
- Recovery may be due to the foot ulcers healing and increased blood flow after plantar electrical stimulation [34].
- According to a study, patients with DPN who received daily electric stimulation for 6 weeks saw a higher improvement in their balance than the group that performed balance exercises [35].
- Electrical noise given directly to sensory neurons has been shown in several studies to improve skin perfusion, repair damaged neurons in DPN patients, and significantly increase the neurons' ability to detect weak signals [34].
- For DPN patients, plantar electrical stimulation enhances plantar sensitivity and postural balance. Ankle and COM sway considerably improved in the intervention group during the 6-week daily study, but there was no improvement in the control group. Their results suggest that protective perception may be improved by current technological advancements. Increasing the mechanoreceptors' effectiveness was one possible tactic [34].

6.2.5.2 Mechanism

Improving mechanoreceptor activity was one effective strategy that may be used. However, damaged Schwann cells can be electrically activated to increase the function of Schwann cells due to the heightened foot feeling and decreased nerve transmission in these patients. Increased skin circulation is linked to an extra electrical stimulation mode; a drop in blood flow might result in oxidative stress or the production of substances that obstruct nerve signal transmission. By releasing vascular endothelial growth factor, electrical stimulation enhances cutaneous flow (VEGE) [34].

6.2.6 PENS (Plantar Electrical Nerve Stimulation)

Research has demonstrated that VEGE stimulates the growth of axons, nerve and cell regeneration, and the proliferation of Schwann cells. Electrical stimulation thereby raises skeletal muscle mRNA activity and VEGE secretion [34].

Electroacupuncture is a technique used to treat the body's energy imbalances by putting needles into various body areas. Transcutaneous or percutaneous electrical nerve stimulation, also known as TENS or PENS, has been used to treat peripheral neuropathy-related pain and suffering besides activating the spinal cord. PENS is a novel form of electro analgesic therapy that combines electroacupuncture and TENS by stimulating peripheral sensory nerves in the region of neuropathic pain with needles that resemble acupuncture needles inserted into the skin (Fig. 6.4). The cumulative benefits of PENS suggest long-term benefits that align with the findings of a 1996 study by Mo et al. that used TENS in conjunction with electroacupuncture in animal models of DPN [36].

Two possibilities have been proposed; however, the exact mechanism underlying the analgesic benefits of PENS use is still unknown: either neuronal regulation or higher concentrations of opioid-like chemicals (endorphin, dynorphin, and enkephalin) in the central nervous system [36].

6.2.6.1 Mechanism

For individuals with DPN, electroacupuncture is a beneficial and secure kind of treatment. The main mechanism is that by dramatically changing blood flow to central endorphins like beta and dynorphin, electroporation raises the tolerance for pain. Increased flux via the polyol pathway, glycation and advanced glycation end products, oxidative stress, protein kinase C activity, and inflammatory processes are a few of the recovery mechanisms linked to electroacupuncture. Conversely, peripheral nerve receptors, pain relief, and cutaneous reinnervation are benefits of electroacupuncture recovery. Moreover, it has been documented that changes in central endorphins like beta or dynorphin cause electroacupuncture to change blood flow. Following therapy, improvements were seen in the following areas: motor efficiency, plantar sensation, life satisfaction, physical activity, discomfort, postural stability, and sleep quality [36].

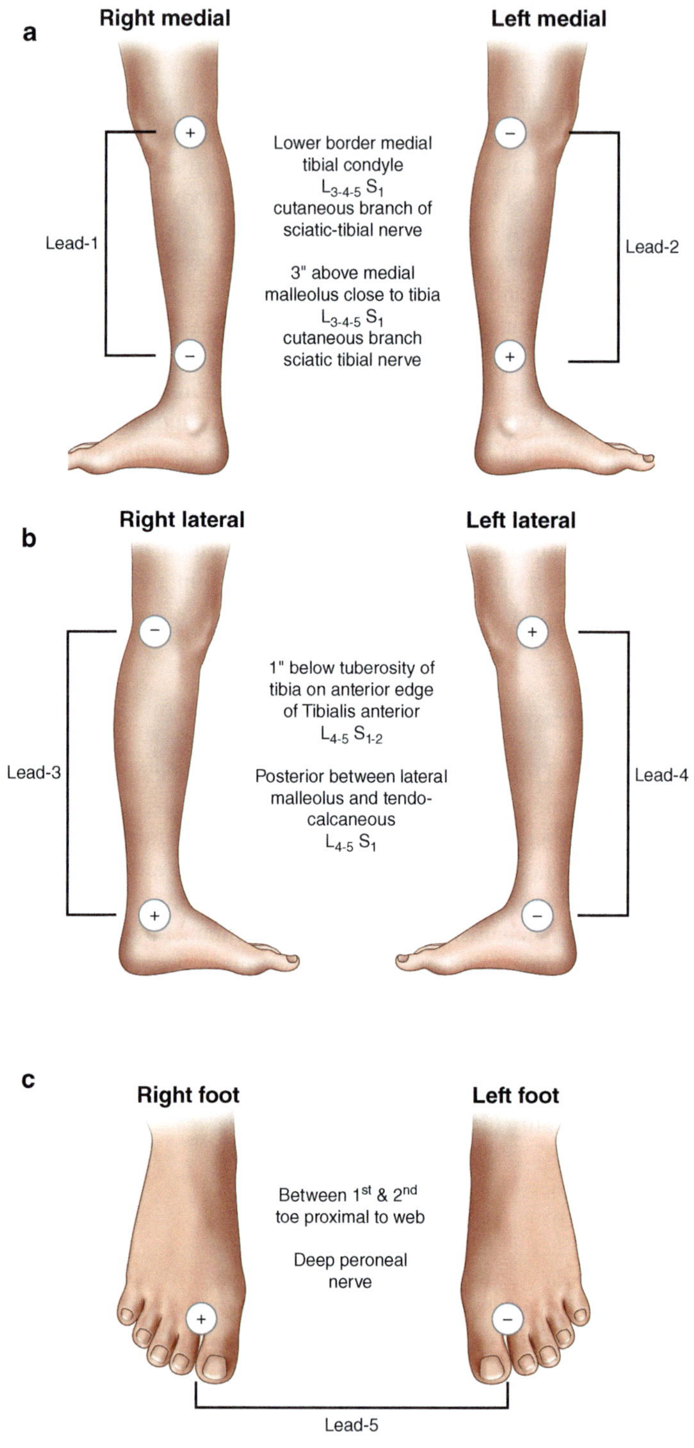

Fig. 6.4 Neuropathic pain treated by PENS electroanalgesia. The placements of the needles for every positive and negative pair [36]

6.3 Other Interventions

6.3.1 (Pulsed Electromagnetic Field) PEMF

Low-frequency electromagnetic field, often known as pulsed electromagnetic field (PEMF), is thought to be a safe adjunctive treatment for DPN patients. Pulsed electromagnetic fields (PEMF), which have analgesic, neuro stimulatory, trophic, and vasoactive effects, are one method that is currently of clinical interest [37].

6.3.1.1 Treatment Procedure

Patient with DPN get treatment using pulsed electromagnetic fields (ASA Easy terza series; Italy). Every patient will put in a supine position, which is a nice and relaxing position.

- The appliance's main electrical connection was at 230 V. The solenoid was programmed to cover the lower leg for 20 min at a frequency of 50 Hz and an intensity of 20 G.
- •Thrice week, every day for 4 weeks, the treatment was administered [38].

6.3.1.1.1 Effects of PEMF in DPN

- PEMF therapy may be able to control nerve impulse and neuropathic pain. Positive changes following treatment sessions may be caused by a reduction in endo neural hypoxia, perineural oedema, peripheral nerve ischemia, and enhanced microcirculation [37].
- The perineurial basement membrane is enlarged and endoneurial capillaries in peripheral nerves of diabetics are thickened, which may account for the PEMF group's better peroneal nerve distal latency and nerve conduction velocity (NCV). Diabetics may experience endoneurial metabolic disturbances due to a permeability issue at the blood nerve or blood perineurial barrier, which could potentially result in neuropathy.
- PEMF reverses the damage that causes peripheral neuropathy by focusing on improved circulation, anti-inflammatory benefits, pain alleviation, and the restoration of normal nerve conduction
- The recent discovery that PEMF influences both nerve regeneration in vivo and neurite formation in vitro.
- Few studies have been conducted on PEMF treatment for diabetic peripheral neuropathy in the literature, but those that have are consistent with the current findings. In one such study, PEMF significantly improved peroneal nerve conduction velocity (m/s) and significantly reduced pain intensity in patients with diabetic neuropathy. The study examined the effects of PEMF on pain and motor nerve conduction velocity (NCV).

- Prior research has demonstrated that PEMFs can influence certain aspects of nerve function in individuals with diabetes and can promote nerve development, regeneration, and functional restoration of nerves in animal models of nerve illness.
- The fundamental function of PEMF is to cause a physiological response, such as cell growth, which serves as an explanation for several pertinent findings. It can increase the number of nerve fibers and, consequently, the amplitude attained in nerve conduction studies by promoting nerve regeneration and hastening recovery in experimentally divided and sutured peroneal nerve.
- PEMF application improves the conductive function of peripheral nerves, the status of 1a afferents, the reflex excitability of functionally varied motor neurons in the spinal cord, and the regression of the primary clinical symptoms of DPN. According to the study's findings, PEMF at 10 Hz has been shown to be therapeutically effective, particularly in the early stages of DPN and in individuals who have had DM for up to 10 years [37].
- This finding supports the theory put forth, according to which magnetic therapy—in which magnets are marketed for their analgesic and energizing properties without side effects—has become one of the fastest-growing alternative therapies. The reduction of pain intensity was better following PEMF treatment. PEMF therapy's analgesic impact may be due to presynaptic inhibition or lower excitability of pain fibers, two physiological processes of pain reduction.
- Additionally, a range of cell types' neurotransmitter surface receptor sites, hormones, and antibodies can all be modulated by PEMF. Chemical processes may be sped up or slowed down as a result of changes in the electron transfer rate that occur during the electron exchange between single molecules.
- Increased activity of damaged small-diameter regenerating fibers, which fire quickly and at unusually low thresholds, is most likely the source of the discomfort. The pericellular and cellular microenvironments are altered by the PEMF's effects on diabetes neurons and the cell membrane of cutaneous nociceptors [37].

PEMF has the potential to be a useful therapeutic method for treating painful diabetic neuropathy since it can alter peripheral nerve function's electrical characteristics and pain perception [39].

6.3.2 Stable Galvanization (SG)

SG is typically given once daily for 20 min, with the electrodes typically positioned longitudinally and descendental down both legs at an intensity of 0.1–0.5 mA/cm^2, depending on the subjective feelings of the patients. The electrodes are rectangular in shape [39].

Hyperaemia in the deeper tissues and epidermis is a sign of SG's analgesic effects. The gate control mechanism, which entails SG's impact on cutaneous sensory endings to inhibit pain in the spinal cord's posterior horns by releasing endogenous opioids, is one reason for the reduction in pain [39].

6.3.3 Monochromatic Infrared Photo Energy (MIRE)

MIRE is a crucial DPN treatment modality that improves muscle power, sensitivity, and nerve conduction velocity (NCV) while also relieving discomfort and neural function that is lost in DPN. MIRE causes the blood arteries in the feet to dilate, which promotes the healing of diabetic foot ulcers by raising the concentration of NO in the blood. Low-level exposure to red and near-IR light triggers the release of NO, and MIRE tends to accelerate healing at sites where the MIRE pad is located. It has been shown that light energy is primarily consumed in the mitochondria by endogenous chromophores and used to synthesize ATP, which is then used to drive metabolic processes necessary for the repair or regeneration of cell and tissue components [40].

6.4 Conclusion

In conclusion, there are several electrotherapy modalities that can be used to manage painful diabetic neuropathy (DPN), and each has a unique mechanism of action that may provide advantages. Both pulsed electromagnetic stimulation (PEMF) and high-frequency transcutaneous electrical nerve stimulation (TENS) show potential in regulating the sensory and motor systems, possibly reducing pain and enhancing nerve function. Adjuvant therapies such as low-power laser therapy and electromagnetic fields are beneficial because they promote enhanced microcirculation, ulcer healing, and decreased inflammation and swelling. Additionally, transcranial direct current stimulation (tDCS), spinal cord stimulation, and repetitive transcranial magnetic stimulation (rTMS) are state-of-the-art techniques for treating neuropathic pain. When these several approaches are combined into comprehensive treatment plans, people with diabetic peripheral neuropathy may experience an improvement in their quality of life.

References

1. Hicks CW, Selvin E. Epidemiology of peripheral neuropathy and lower extremity disease in diabetes. Curr Diab Rep. 2019;19(10):86.
2. Sloan G, Shillo P, Selvarajah D, Wu J, Wilkinson ID, Tracey I, Anand P, Tesfaye S. A new look at painful diabetic neuropathy. Diabetes Res Clin Pract. 2018;144:177–91.
3. Bernetti A, Agostini F, de Sire A, Mangone M, Tognolo L, Di Cesare A, Ruiu P, Paolucci T, Invernizzi M, Paoloni M. Neuropathic pain and rehabilitation: a systematic review of international guidelines. Diagnostics (Basel). 2021;11(1):74.
4. Karypidou M, Lytras D, Kottaras A, Iakovidis P, Tsimerakis AF, Georgios L. Effects of electrotherapy in neuropathic pain management in patients with diabetic peripheral neuropathy: a narrative review. IJACM. 2021;4(2):35–8.

5. Pieber K, Herceg M, Paternostro-Sluga T. Electrotherapy for the treatment of painful diabetic peripheral neuropathy: a review. J Rehabil Med. 2010;42(4):289–95. https://doi.org/10.2340/16501977-0554.
6. Gibson W, Wand BM, O'Connell NE. Transcutaneous electrical nerve stimulation (TENS) for neuropathic pain in adults. Cochrane Database Syst Rev. 2017;9(9):CD011976. https://doi.org/10.1002/14651858.CD011976.pub2.
7. Mokhtari T, Ren Q, Li N, Wang F, Bi Y, Hu L. Transcutaneous electrical nerve stimulation in relieving neuropathic pain: basic mechanisms and clinical applications. Curr Pain Headache Rep. 2020;24:1–14.
8. Gossrau G, Wähner M, Kuschke M, Konrad B, Reichmann H, Wiedemann B, Sabatowski R. Microcurrent transcutaneous electric nerve stimulation in painful diabetic neuropathy: a randomized placebo-controlled study. Pain Med. 2011;12(6):953–60.
9. Jin DM, Xu Y, Geng DF, Yan TB. Effect of transcutaneous electrical nerve stimulation on symptomatic diabetic peripheral neuropathy: a meta-analysis of randomized controlled trials. Diabetes Res Clin Pract. 2010;89(1):10–5.
10. Chesterton LS, Foster NE, Wright CC, Baxter GD, Barlas P. Effects of TENS frequency, intensity and stimulation site parameter manipulation on pressure pain thresholds in healthy human subjects. Pain. 2003;106(1-2):73–80.
11. Johnson M. Transcutaneous Electrical Nerve Stimulation: mechanisms, clinical application and evidence. Rev Pain. 2007;1(1):7–11.
12. Melzack R, Wall PD. Pain mechanisms: a new theory. Science. 1965;150(3699):971–9.
13. Liebano RE, Rakel B, Vance CGT, Walsh DM, Sluka KA. An investigation of the development of analgesic tolerance to TENS in humans. Pain. 2011;152(2):335–42.
14. Wutz A, Melcher D, Samaha J. Frequency modulation of neural oscillations according to visual task demands. Proc Natl Acad Sci USA. 2018;115(6):1346–51.
15. Ploner M, Sorg C, Gross J. Brain rhythms of pain. Trends Cogn Sci. 2017;21(2):100–10.
16. Kalra A, Urban MO, Sluka KA. Blockade of opioid receptors in rostral ventral medulla prevents antihyperalgesia produced by transcutaneous electrical nerve stimulation (TENS). J Pharmacol Exp Ther. 2001;298(1):257–63.
17. Hashmi JT, Huang YY, Osmani BZ, Sharma SK, Naeser MA, Hamblin MR. Role of low-level laser therapy in neurorehabilitation. PM R J Inj Funct Rehabil. 2010;2(12 Suppl 2):S292–305.
18. Robijns J, Censabella S, Bulens P, Maes A, Mebis J. The use of low-level light therapy in supportive care for patients with breast cancer: review of the literature. Lasers Med Sci. 2017;32(1):229–42.
19. Lins RD, Dantas EM, Lucena KC, Catão MH, Granville-Garcia AF, Carvalho Neto LG. Biostimulation effects of low-power laser in the repair process. An Bras Dermatol. 2010;85(6):849–55.
20. Schindl A, Schindl M, Pernerstorfer-Schön H, Schindl L. Low-intensity laser therapy: a review. J Investig Med. 2000;48(5):312–26.
21. Anju M, Maiya AG, Hande M. Low level laser therapy for the patients with painful diabetic peripheral neuropathy—a systematic review. Diabetes Metab Syndr. 2019;13(4):2667–70.
22. Abdel-Wahhab KG, Daoud EM, El Gendy A, Mourad HH, Mannaa FA, Saber MM. Efficiencies of low-level laser therapy (LLLT) and gabapentin in the management of peripheral neuropathy: diabetic neuropathy. Appl Biochem Biotechnol. 2018;186:161–73.
23. Atiaa AG, Balah OFA, Mostafa KHA, Abas DN, El Wahab HHA. Effect of low level laser therapy on nerve conduction velocity in diabetic neuropathic patients: a randomized controlled trial. Ann RSCB. 2021;25(3):355–62.
24. Rahin H, Jackson WS, Thordstein M. Effect of transcutaneous spinal direct current stimulation in patients with painful polyneuropathy and influence of possible predictors of efficacy including BDNF polymorphism: a randomized, sham-controlled crossover study. Brain Sci. 2023;13(2):229.

25. Filipas L, Gallo G, Meloni A, Luzi L, Codella R. Effects of bilateral dorsolateral prefrontal cortex high-definition transcranial direct-current stimulation on time-trial performance in cyclists with type 1 diabetes mellitus. Brain Stimul. 2022;15(5):1292–9.
26. ElSayed SH, Moawd SA, Abdelbasset WK. Assessment of the quality of life following transcranial direct current stimulation in patients with diabetic peripheral neuropathy. J Adv Pharm Educ Res. 2020;10(1):9–13.
27. Alipour A, Mohammadi R. Evaluation of the separate and combined effects of anodal tDCS over the M1 and F3 regions on pain relief in patients with type-2 diabetes suffering from neuropathic pain. Neurosci Lett. 2024;818:137554.
28. Ferreira G, Silva-Filho E, de Oliveira A, de Lucena C, Lopes J, Pegado R. Transcranial direct current stimulation improves quality of life and physical fitness in diabetic polyneuropathy: a pilot double blind randomized controlled trial. J Diabetes Metab Disord. 2020;19:327–35.
29. Tsai YY, Wu WT, Han DS, Mezian K, Ricci V, Özçakar L, Chang KV. Application of repetitive transcranial magnetic stimulation in neuropathic pain: a narrative review. Life. 2023;13(2):258.
30. Seminowicz DA, Moayedi M. The dorsolateral prefrontal cortex in acute and chronic pain. J Pain. 2017;18(9):1027–35.
31. Chu CS, Li CT, Brunoni AR, Yang FC, Tseng PT, Tu YK, Stubbs B, Carvalho AF, Thompson T, Rajji TK, Yeh TC, Tsai CK, Chen TY, Li DJ, Hsu CW, Wu YC, Yu CL, Liang CS. Cognitive effects and acceptability of non-invasive brain stimulation on Alzheimer's disease and mild cognitive impairment: a component network meta-analysis. J Neurol Neurosurg Psychiatry. 2021;92(2):195–203.
32. Jiang X, Yan W, Wan R, Lin Y, Zhu X, Song G, Zheng K, Wang Y, Wang X. Effects of repetitive transcranial magnetic stimulation on neuropathic pain: a systematic review and meta-analysis. Neurosci Biobehav Rev. 2022 Jan;132:130–41. https://doi.org/10.1016/j.neubiorev.2021.11.037.
33. Yang S, Kwak SG, Choi GS, Chang MC. Short-term effect of repetitive transcranial magnetic stimulation on diabetic peripheral neuropathic pain. Pain Physician. 2022;25(2):E203.
34. Najafi B, Talal TK, Grewal GS, Menzies R, Armstrong DG, Lavery LA. Using plantar electrical stimulation to improve postural balance and plantar sensation among patients with diabetic peripheral neuropathy: a randomized double blinded study. J Diabetes Sci Technol. 2017;11(4):693–701.
35. Grewal GS, Schwenk M, Lee-Eng J, Parvaneh S, Bharara M, Menzies RA, Talal TK, Armstrong DG, Najafi B. Sensor-based interactive balance training with visual joint movement feedback for improving postural stability in diabetics with peripheral neuropathy: a randomized controlled trial. Gerontology. 2015;61(6):567–74.
36. Jahantigh Akbari N, Hosseinifar M, Naimi SS, Mikaili S, Rahbar S. The efficacy of physiotherapy interventions in mitigating the symptoms and complications of diabetic peripheral neuropathy: a systematic review. J Diabetes Metab Disord. 2020;19(2):1995–2004. https://doi.org/10.1007/s40200-020-00652-8.
37. Mohamed RA, Abdallah GA, Abdeen HA, Nassif AA. Influence of low-level laser therapy versus pulsed electromagnetic field on diabetic peripheral neuropathy. Phys Ther Rehab. 2017;4(1):17.
38. Mirkovic VB, Banjac L, Dasic Z, Dapcevic M. Non-pharmacological treatment of diabetic polyneuropathy by pulse electromagnetic field. HealthMED. 2012;6:1291–5.
39. Grbović V, Stefanović S, Đukić S, Nurković J, Zdravković PN, Parezanović IK, et al. The effects of the physical procedures in patients with diabetic neuropathy. Vojnosanit Pregl. 2019;76(8):787–94.
40. Sahier OEK, Yousief EM, Rabab AM, El Gendy MH, El Khalek A, Elsiofy Mohamed MM. Effect of monochromatic infrared energy light versus laser therapy in diabetic peripheral neuropathy. Med J Cairo Univ. 2020;88(3):521–8.

Chapter 7
Nerve-Targeted Rehabilitation Approaches for Diabetic Peripheral Neuropathy

Akanksha Saxena and Kanika

Contents

A. Saxena (✉) · Kanika
Department of Neurological Physiotherapy, Maharishi Markandeshwar Institute of Physiotherapy & Rehabilitation, MM(DU), Ambala, Haryana, India

© The Author(s), under exclusive license to Springer Nature Singapore Pte Ltd. 2024

M. Goyal, K. Goyal (eds.), *Rehabilitation in Diabetic Peripheral Neuropathy*,
https://doi.org/10.1007/978-981-97-9290-0_7

7.1 Introduction

Worldwide 451 million persons are living with diabetes mellitus which is expected to rise to 639 million by 2045 [1]. Diabetes peripheral neuropathy is a most severe complication of diabetes mellitus accounting for almost 90% of the cases and is a leading cause of foot amputations [2, 3]. Diabetes mellitus Type 1 and Type 2 both are affected with higher incidence in type 2 patients [4]. Presentation of diabetic peripheral neuropathy (DPN) is usually bilateral and symmetrical progressing from distally to proximally involving both motor and sensory components [4]. Pain is usually presented as dysesthesia due to small-nerve fibers involvement and sometimes as mechanical allodynia and hyperalgesia, whereas numbness and sensory loss can be due to large nerve fiber involvement [4, 5].

Several factors cause development of DPN, ranging from chronic uncontrolled hyperglycemia, neural inflammation, and microvascular insufficiency all causing decrease in neural blood flow and later resulting in ischemia of nerves. Increasing pro-inflammatory mediators also cause sensitization of nerve endings leading to mechanical hypersensitivity [3, 6]. Dyslipidemia and decreased neuronal responsiveness are primary contributors to DPN. Additionally, a decrease in both insulin and C-peptide levels plays a notable role in the development of DPN [7]. Figure 7.1 shows the difference between a peripheral healthy nerve and a peripheral nerve in cases of diabetic peripheral neuropathy.

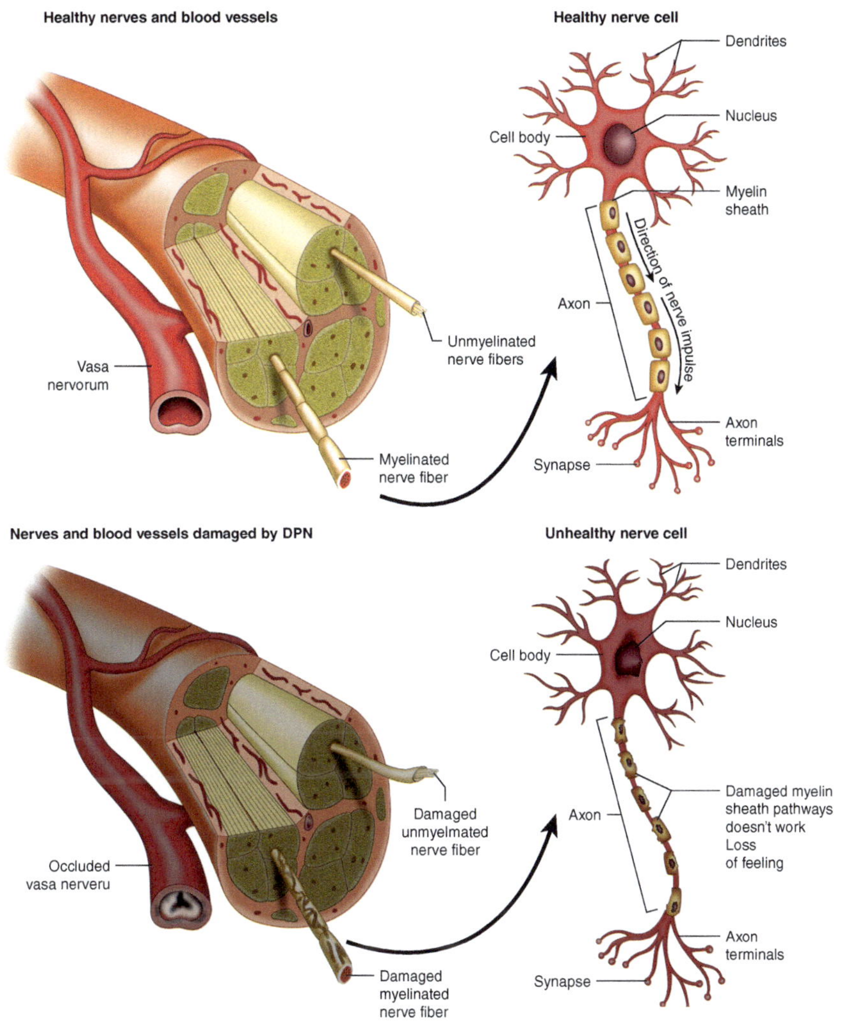

Fig. 7.1 Comparison of a healthy nerve and a DPN nerve

7.2 Pathomechanical/Pathophysiological Responses of Nerve in DPN

Various factors are associated with the nerve degeneration in patients with DPN [8]. The most widely proposed mechanism is shown in Fig. 7.2.

The management of DPN is rather complex as the chosen therapy must work upon reducing the neural inflammation and nerve degeneration while simultaneously inducing nerve regeneration. According to American diabetes association guidelines, lifestyle changes and glycemic control can prevent and halt the progression of DPN [9]. Earlier researches also suggested that exercise can halt or alter the symptoms of DPN [5, 6]. Zilliox et al. in his review done in 2019 stated that physical activity and dietary changes can also modify the course and symptoms of DPN in human and animal models. In another randomized controlled trial on participants with diabetic peripheral neuropathy, a submaximal aerobic exercise regime of 4 h/week improved nerve conduction velocity of peroneal nerve suggesting improvements in both motor and sensory parameters in individuals with DPN [10, 11].

Elevated reaction time and diminished proprioception lead to instability in posture and impairments in balance. Consequently, individuals with DPN encounter challenges in maintaining equilibrium, even with their eyes open, which increases the risk of falls. DPN has been linked to persistent disability caused by foot ulcers, amputations, balance issues, unstable gait, and fall-related injuries. Approximately, 20–30% of individuals with DPN suffer from neuropathic pain [12].

The most novel technique which is recently being used to modify or treat the symptoms of DPN is the use of neural mobilization or nerve massage/neurodynamics and neuromuscular taping.

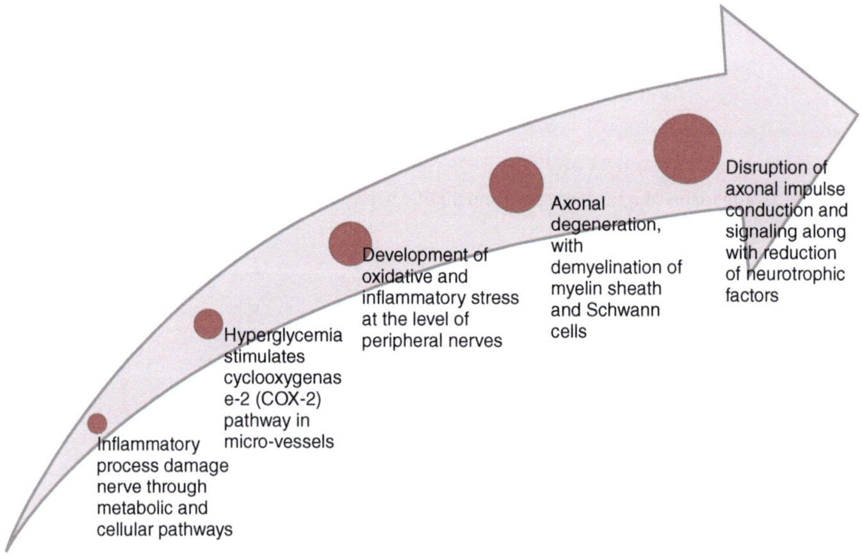

Fig. 7.2 Pathomechanical and pathophysiological responses of a nerve in DPN

7.3 Neurodynamics

Neurodynamics is the term coined by Michael Shacklock and it links mechanics, physiology, and function of the musculoskeletal system with the neural system. It was originated from the concept of "Adverse Mechanical tension" given by Breig and Marions [13]. As per Coppieters and Butler: "This clinical concept utilizes movement to evaluate heightened mechanosensitivity of the nervous system and to rejuvenate homeostasis within and surrounding the nervous system" [14].

According to Butler [15], the central and peripheral nervous systems (PNS) are regarded as one system supported by three dimensions: first is chemical continuity, which is upheld by both central and peripheral neurotransmitters as well as axoplasmic flow, ensuring the proper guidance of nutrients from the nervous system into the axon, second is mechanical continuity which is evidenced by the transmission of forces and movements facilitated by connective tissue sheaths surrounding nerve cells and the last one is electrical continuity, which is upheld by neurons and facilitates transmission from one part of the body to another. Consequently, it is thought that following a central or PNS damage, tension increases and impairs the nervous system's ability to move freely and function normally [15]. Thus it proves that mechanical and physiological events occurring in the nervous system anywhere are interdependent on each other and can affect the tension in other parts too of the nervous system [16]. The surrounding tissues around the nerves are called as "mechanical interface," i.e., the nerve bed, joints, muscles, fascia, etc. Any inflammatory changes occurring in the nerve can lead to changes in the mechanical interface and vice versa leading to intraneural fibrosis [17–19].

Neural mobilization is a technique deduced from the above concept to treat adverse mechanical tension, the goal of which is to place the neuroaxis in tension through rhythmic repetitive postures of the limb. It can reinstate the compressive, sliding, and elongation ability of the neural tissues [14, 20] by facilitating gliding of the nerve, reducing nerve adhesions, enhancing neural blood flow, dispersing noxious fluids and improving axoplasmic flow [21]. Neural mobilization has been explored in almost all conditions, be it in stroke and spinal cord injury in reducing spasticity and improving range of motion [22–26] or in radiculopathies and nerve palsies [27].

7.4 Neurodynamics in Diabetic Peripheral Neuropathy

As per the International Association for the study of pain: "neuropathic pain arose due to any pathology in the nervous system." Peripheral neuropathic pain, frequently observed in diabetic DPN, typically manifests as a blend of nerve trunk pain and dysesthetic pain [28]. Nerve trunk pain is a deep aching pain resulting from the increased activity of the sensitized nociceptors within the connective tissue sheaths of the nerves, whereas dysesthetic pain is the result of the damaged or regenerating afferent nerve fibers which generates abnormal impulses leading to mechanical allodynia and hyperalgesia in both human and animal subjects with DPN. This mechanosensitivity is effectively managed by neurodynamic techniques as seen in reviews done by Ellis and Hing and Nee and Butler et al. [21, 29]. Neural mobilizations in rat models have been known to reduce not only the symptoms of mechanical allodynia but also delays development of hyperalgesia and allodynia [6, 30]. Even it delays nerve degeneration by a single session of neural mobilization for atleast 48 h and promotes nerve regeneration by increasing nerve growth factors and myelin protein zero and reduced inter-neuronal fibrosis in rats [31, 32]. Nerve Massage along the course of the nerve can reduce the adhesions in the nerve and prevent inter-neuronal fibrosis while maintaining normal vascularity and conduction of the nerve.

7.5 Nerve Massage in DPN

Fluid accumulation in the nerve causes altered nerve mechanics which can be reversed by neural mobilization and nerve massage [33]. In a study by Kumar et al., immediate effects of nerve sliders and nerve massage were observed on vibration perception and heat perception thresholds in individuals with DPN indicating that mechanosensitivity can be reduced by nerve massage and sliders [34]. In another case report, pain and range of motion improved after longitudinal and transverse tibial nerve massage after six sessions in a patient with diabetic peripheral neuropathy [35]. To perform nerve massage effectively, palpation of the nerve along its course and the determination of an abnormal response in terms of hyperalgesia, tenderness or thickening and swelling is a pre-requisite.

7.5.1 Tibial Nerve Massage

Patient Position: Prone lying or side lying with extended knee and limb in neutral position.

Therapist position: On side of the treating limb of the patient.

Procedure: First locate the nerve with the help of the thumb pads, in the middle of the two dimples behind the knee. After palpation of the nerve, apply gentle longitudinal and transverse massage (Fig. 7.3) along the course of the nerve, five times each for 6–6 repetitions [33–35].

7.5.2 Peroneal Nerve Massage

Patient Position: Supine lying with knee flexed in 90 degrees.

Therapist position: In front of the treating limb of the patient.

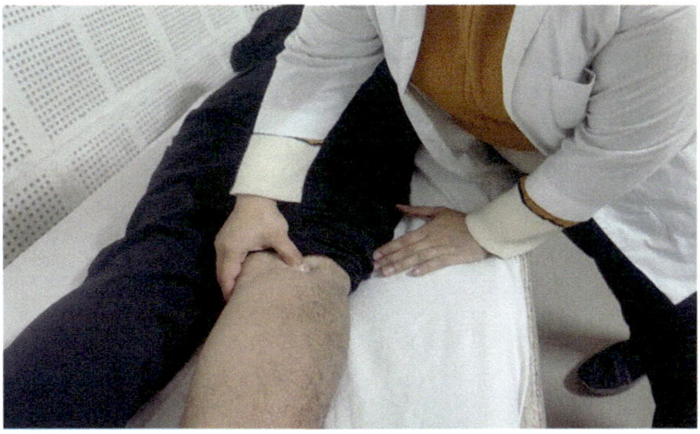

Fig. 7.3 Tibial nerve massage hand placement

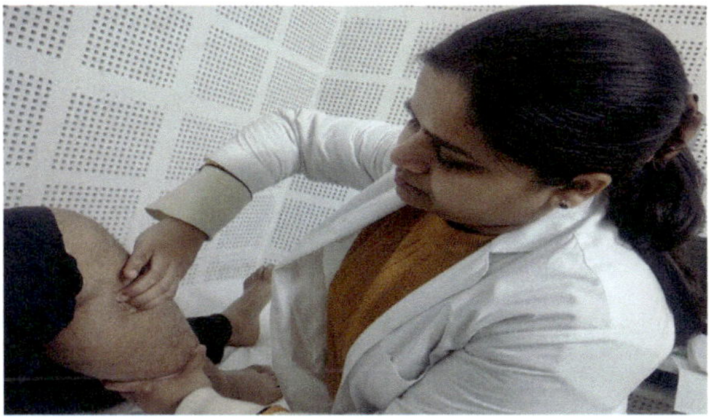

Fig. 7.4 Peroneal nerve massage hand placement

Procedure: First find the head of the fibula of the treated limb and then locate the nerve with the help of the pads of the index and middle finger, horizontally along the neck of the fibula. After palpation of the nerve, apply gentle longitudinal and transverse massage by moving your fingers (Fig. 7.4) along the course of the nerve for five times each massage for 6–6 [34].

7.5.3 *Sural Nerve Massage*

Patient Position: Supine lying with limb in neutral position and leg hanging off the couch.

Therapist position: In front of the treating limb of the patient.

Procedure: First locate the nerve with the help of the thumb and finger pads on the medial aspect of the Achilles tendon as shown in Fig. 7.5. After palpation of the nerve, try rolling your thumb over the nerve then apply gentle longitudinal and transverse massage along the course of the nerve, five times each for 6–6 repetitions [34].

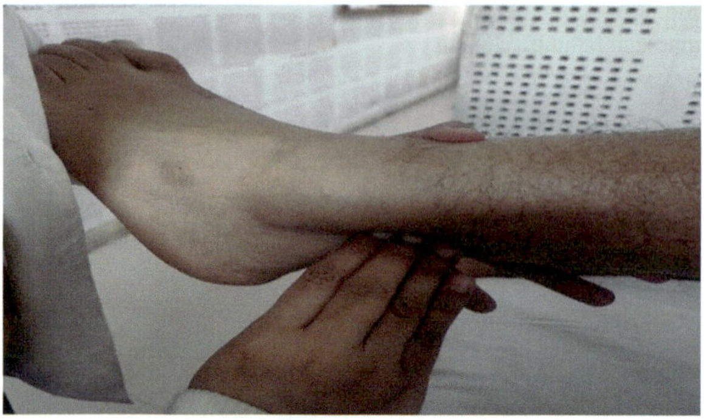
Fig. 7.5 Sural nerve massage hand placement

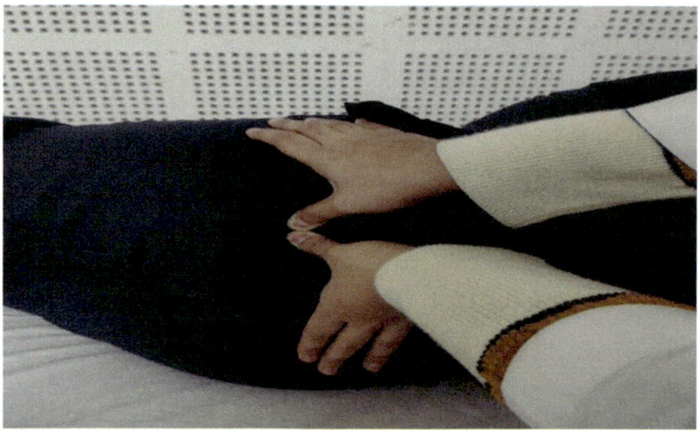
Fig. 7.6 Sciatic nerve massage hand placement

7.5.4 Sciatic Nerve Massage

Patient Position: Side lying with slightly flexed knee of the limb which is facing the ceiling.

Therapist position: Facing the buttocks of the patient.

Procedure: First locate the nerve in the groove made between the posterior aspect of the greater trochanter and lateral aspect of ischial tuberosity as shown in Fig. 7.6. Then locate the nerve with the help of the thumb pads and apply gentle longitudinal and transverse massage by moving your fingers (Fig. 7.6) along the course of the nerve for five times each massage for 6–6 repetitions [34].

7.6 Neural Mobilization in DPN

Two neural mobilization techniques—sliders and tensioners are given by Butler [15] and Shacklock [16]. In sliders, nerve ends move in same direction and it facilitates sliding movement in the neural tissue by loading or tensioning the nerve at one joint while unloading or slacking the nerve at other joint. Tensioners are like the

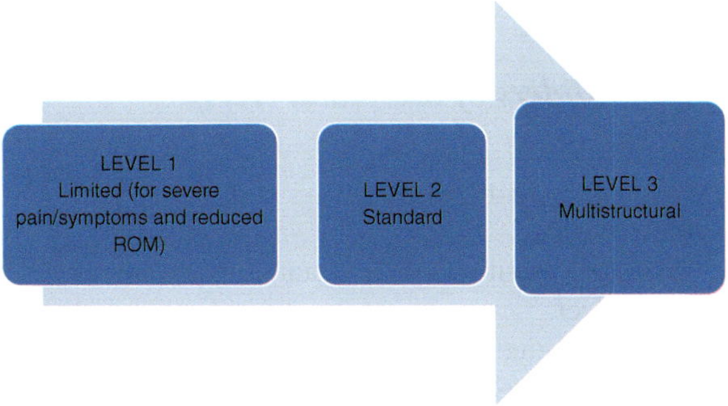

Fig. 7.7 Selection of technique. (Note: Remote sliders simply mean keeping the joints in reduced ROM and sliders will only use joints that are pain free. Given below are all standard sliders in which modifications can be made for remote sliders)

tension testing and they lengthen or create tension in the nerve bed without surpassing the elastic limit of the nerve [14, 36–40]. Pain in DPN is caused mainly due to the development of epineural and endoneuraledema and the lack of lymphatic vessels in endoneurium restricts its drainage. Hence developing a "minicompartment syndrome" within the nerve, this will further cause fibrosis and adhesions thus limiting intrafascicular gliding. According to the cadaveric study done by Brown et al., tensioners performed at ankle of tibial nerve is improving ankle range of motion [41]. The same improvements on ankle ROM were also evident in another study done on DPN [42].

Neural mobilization is contraindicated in cases where severe pain is there or symptoms are progressively deteriorating or psychological or cognitive issues are there with the patient. To select an appropriate technique, first learning the level of techniques is essential (Fig. 7.7). Level 1/ Limited technique are used when pain is severe and take time to settle down and the joints have reduced range of motion. Level 2/ Standard technique are used when pain is between mild to moderate, range of motion is full and symptoms are sort of stable. Level 3/Multistructural technique is used when the problem is Multistructural and involves mechanical interface too i.e. patient having neural and musculoskeletal symptoms too.

- For patients who require Level 1 technique, Remote sliders will be used followed by standard sliders and then tensioners.
- For patients who require Level 2 technique, Standard sliders will be used followed by tensioners.
- For patients who require Level 3 technique, first work will be done on the mechanical interface or the musculoskeletal problem followed by standard sliders and tensioners.

Treatment Parameters

- Technique—Sliders/Tensioners
- Speed—3–4 s/ oscillation
- Repetition—15–20 reps/min
- Duration—30 s to 2 min, 5 sets with 1 min of rest between the sets

7.7 Sliders

7.7.1 Sliders of the Tibial Nerve

Position of patient—Supine, without pillow and hip and pelvis aligned symmetrically.

Therapist position—Stride standing by the side of the couch facing toward the patient's feet.

Hand placement—one hand on the patient's ankle with a distal hand hold keeping ankle in DF/Eversion and other hand supporting over patient's anterior aspect of the knee followed by passive Straight Leg raise to about 35–70 degree of hip flexion in a pain free range.

Procedure: Therapist will first load the nerve at ankle with Dorsiflexion/Eversion and keeping the knee in flexion (unloading the nerve) and then smoothly moving the ankle in Plantarflexion/Inversion (unloading the nerve) with Knee in extension(loading the nerve) [33, 35, 42, 43]. Refer Fig. 7.8.

7.7.2 Sliders of the Peroneal Nerve

Position of patient—Supine, without pillow and hip and pelvis aligned symmetrically.

Therapist position—Stride standing by the side of the couch facing toward the patient's feet and leaning to hold ankle with hand and supporting by elbow.

Hand placement—one hand on the patient's ankle with a distal hand hold keeping ankle in PF/inversion and other hand supporting over patient's anterior aspect of the knee followed by passive Straight leg raise to about 35–70 degree of hip flexion in a pain free range.

Procedure: Therapist will first load the nerve at ankle with plantarflexion/inversion and keeping the knee in flexion (unloading the nerve) and then smoothly moving the ankle in dorsiflexion/eversion (unloading the nerve) with knee in extension (loading the nerve) [42, 43]. Refer Fig. 7.9.

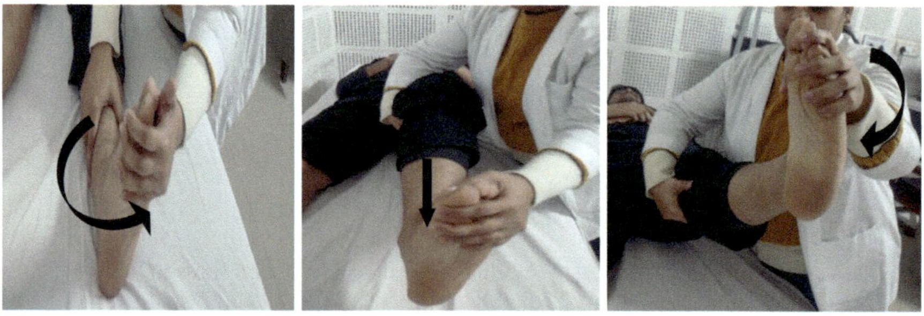

Fig. 7.8 Sliders of tibial nerve

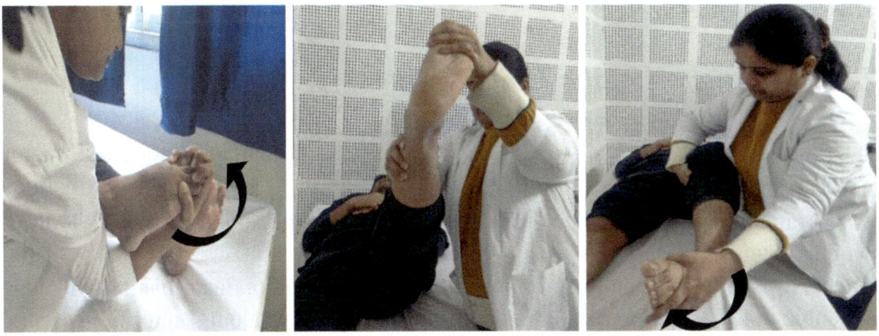

Fig. 7.9 Sliders of peroneal nerve

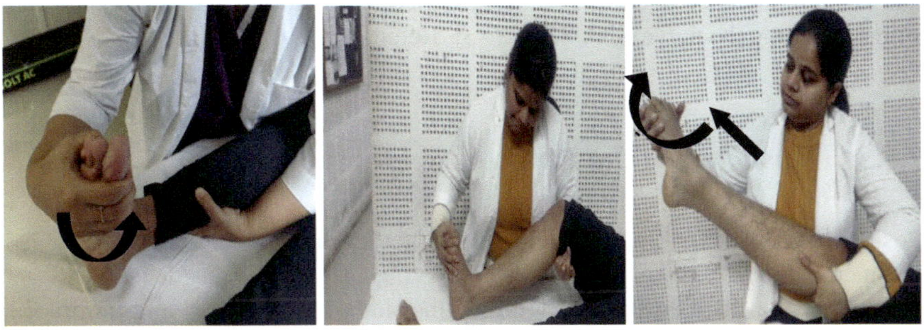

Fig. 7.10 Sliders of sural nerve

7.7.3 Sliders of the Sural Nerve

Position of patient—Supine, without pillow and hip and pelvis aligned symmetrically.

Therapist position—Stride standing by the side of the couch facing toward the patient's feet and leaning to hold ankle with hand and supporting by elbow.

Hand placement—one hand(distal) on the patient's ankle medially around the foot keeping ankle in DF/Inversion and other hand passes medial around tibia and fibula supporting over patient's anterior aspect of the knee followed by passive straight leg raise to about 35–70 degree of hip flexion in a pain free range.

Procedure: Therapist will first load the nerve at ankle with Dorsiflexion/Inversion and keeping the knee in flexion (unloading the nerve) and then smoothly moving the ankle in Plantarflexion/Eversion (unloading the nerve) with knee in extension (loading the nerve) [43]. Refer Fig. 7.10.

7.8 Tensioners

7.8.1 Tensioners of the Tibial Nerve

Position of patient—Supine, without pillow and hip and pelvis aligned symmetrically.

Therapist position—Stride standing by the side of the couch facing toward the patient's feet.

Hand placement—one hand on the patient's ankle with a distal hand hold keeping ankle in DF/Eversion and other hand supporting over patient's anterior aspect of the knee followed by passive Straight Leg raise to about 35–70 degree of hip flexion in a pain free range.

Procedure: Therapist will first load the nerve at ankle with dorsiflexion/eversion and keeping the knee fixed in extension, moving the ankle in plantarflexion/inversion (unloading the nerve) [33, 35, 42, 43]. Refer Fig. 7.11.

7.8.2 Tensioners of the Peroneal Nerve

Position of patient—Supine, without pillow and hip and pelvis aligned symmetrically.

Therapist position—Stride standing by the side of the couch facing toward the patient's feet and leaning to hold ankle with hand and supporting by elbow.

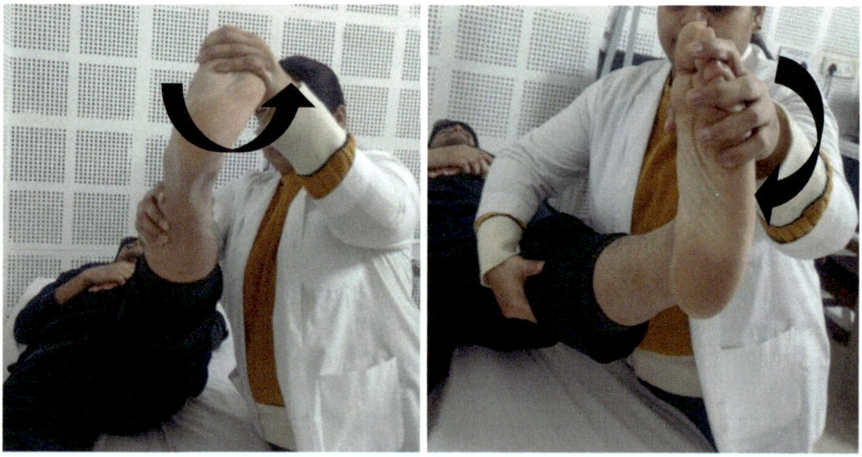

Fig. 7.11 Tensioners of tibial nerve

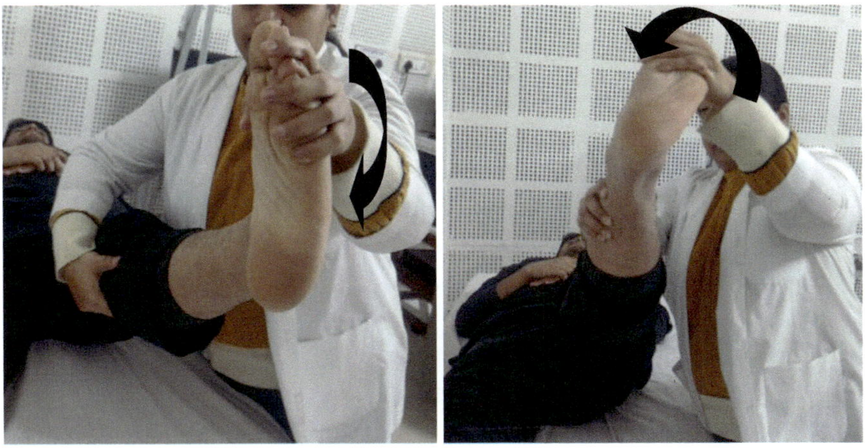

Fig. 7.12 Tensioners of peroneal nerve

Hand placement—one hand on the patient's ankle with a distal hand hold keeping ankle in PF/Inversion and other hand supporting over patient's anterior aspect of the knee followed by passive Straight leg raise to about 35–70 degree of hip flexion in a pain free range.

Procedure: Therapist will first load the nerve at ankle with plantarflexion/inversion and keeping the knee fixed in extension, moving the ankle in dorsiflexion/eversion (unloading the nerve) [33, 43]. Refer Fig. 7.12.

7.8.3 *Tensioners of the Sural Nerve*

Position of patient—Supine, without pillow and hip and pelvis aligned symmetrically.

Therapist position—Stride standing by the side of the couch facing toward the patient's feet and leaning to hold ankle with hand and supporting by elbow.

Hand placement—one hand (distal) on the patient's ankle medially around the foot keeping ankle in DF/Inversion and other hand passes medial around tibia and fibula supporting over patient's anterior aspect of the knee followed by passive Straight Leg raise to about 35–70 degree of hip flexion in a pain free range.

Procedure: Therapist will first load the nerve at ankle with dorsiflexion/inversion and keeping the knee fixed in extension, moving the ankle in plantarflexion/eversion (loading the nerve) [43]. Refer Fig. 7.13.

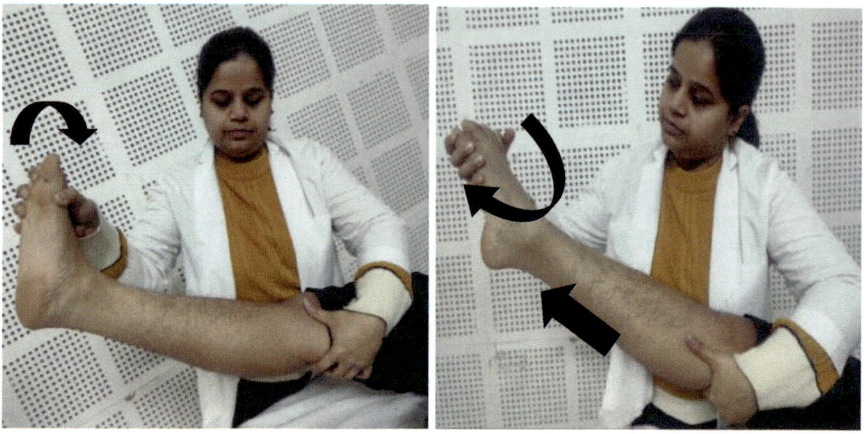

Fig. 7.13 Tensioners of sural nerve

7.9 Neuromuscular Taping in DPN

Taping has been a known rehabilitation approach to treat symptoms associated with diabetic peripheral neuropathy (DPN). Different applications of taping are used in the literature to treat various symptoms of DPN. In physiotherapy, two types of tapes are used for rehabilitation. One type of taping utilizes the use of stretching, such as kinesio taping or functional tape, which uses a specific compression or certain amount of stretching. The second type of taping, i.e., neuromuscular taping (NMT), uses non-stretching tape and includes the application of a tape with no stretch in it [44, 45].

NMT is a newly emerging treatment concept of *decompression* taping developed by **David Leonard Blow** in 2003. NMT is a type of adhesive tape made up of high-quality cotton with an acrylic adhesive layer. It is breathable and water-resistant. It is a non-pharmacological, non-invasive treatment approach in which a tape is applied to the affected area to improve peripheral blood circulation. It is applied to the stretched skin without any tension in it. This application will allow wrinkling of the skin, which further increases with movement, thereby inducing effects on the underlying body tissue [46].

7.10 Physiological Effects of NMT

The application of neuromuscular taping (NMT) appears to alter the sensorimotor integration process. This process involves the stimulation or activation of cutaneous mechanoceptors [47]. It is theorized that NMT has the capability to activate these

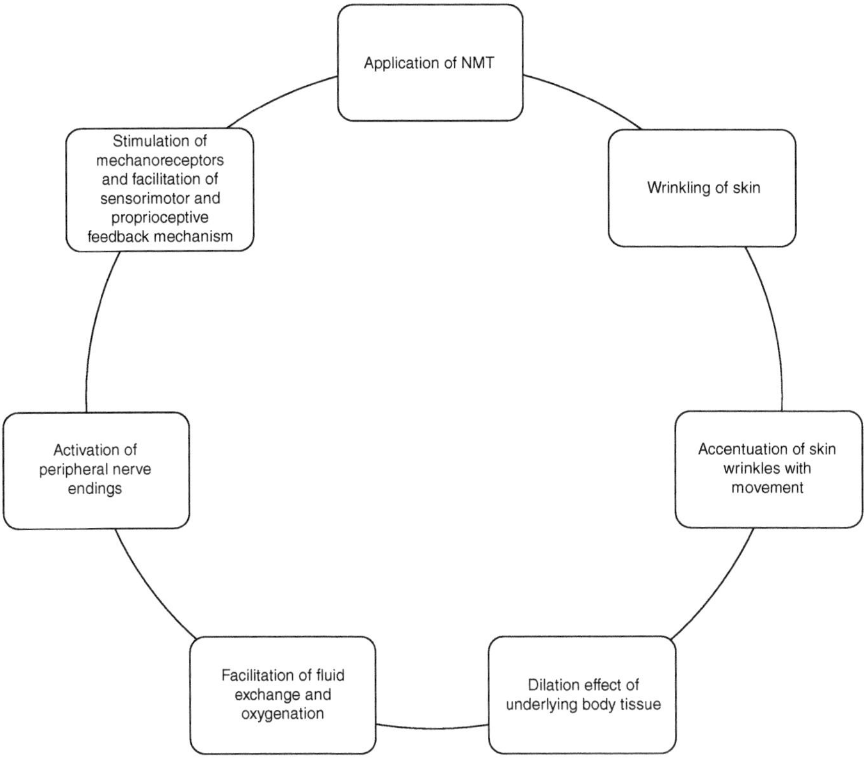

Fig. 7.14 Pathophysiological effect of NMT

cutaneous mechanoceptors, which, in turn, generate nerve impulses in response to mechanical loads such as touch, pressure, vibration, stretch, and itch, leading to deformation. When appropriately stimulated, these receptors induce local depolarization, initiating nerve impulses along afferent fibers directed toward the central nervous system [48]. Refer to Fig. 7.14.

NMT is specifically designed to induce a dilation effect, aiming to enhance peripheral circulation. Its stimulatory impact extends across various tissues in the body, encompassing muscles, fascia, tendons, nerve tissue, lymphatic vessels, and blood vessels. When applied, NMT creates surface skin wrinkles, facilitating passive skin stretching. When the tape is applied without tension, generating an elongation force, it aids in both muscle contraction and relaxation [44].

NMT has been proven to promote lymphatic drainage and improved blood flow through a superficial pumping mechanism. Additionally, NMT generates mechanical stimuli that diminish pressure on the mechanoreceptors, thereby modifying the transmission of painful stimulus. This modification takes place by stimulating Aβ fibers in the inhibitory neurons located within the substantia gelatinosa of Rolando (SGR) in the posterior horn of the spinal cord, thereby inhibiting the pain signal transmission. Application of NMT acts as a mechanical stimulus that aligns with the principles of the Gate Control Theory, concurrently fostering neuron repair by improving fluid exchange and providing nourishment to the vasa nervorum [49].

7.11 NMT in DPN

Muchsin et al., in their study, found significant improvement in pain scores. NMT applied at bilateral foot for a total of 4 weeks, together with oral supplementation of vitamin B complex, as compared to the conventional group, who only received vitamin B complex in patients with painful distal symmetrical polyneuropathy [49].

Susanti and Arofiati found that the application of neuromuscular taping was effective in improving the values of ankle-brachial index (ABI) with a mean of 12.14% in patients with diabetes mellitus [46].

Thakur and Goyal developed a protocol to improve proprioception and balance in patients with DPN. The presence of wrinkles produced by the application of NMT has a positive effect on sensorimotor and proprioceptive functions. It is well established in the literature that impaired proprioception is a contributing factor for affected balance and impaired postural stability [50].

Thakur and Goyal introduced the concept of applying NMT to the four most affected soft tissues in patients with DPN: tibialis anterior, tibialis posterior, peroneus longus, and transverse arch of the foot [50].

7.12 NMT for Transverse Arch of Foot

Position of patient—Supine with lower limbs in neutral position at hip, knee, and ankle.

Therapist position—standing by the side of the patient.

Procedure: The tape will commence anterior to the lateral malleolus, extend beneath the plantar aspect of the foot, and lift the transverse arch of the foot without applying tension. Refer Fig. 7.15.

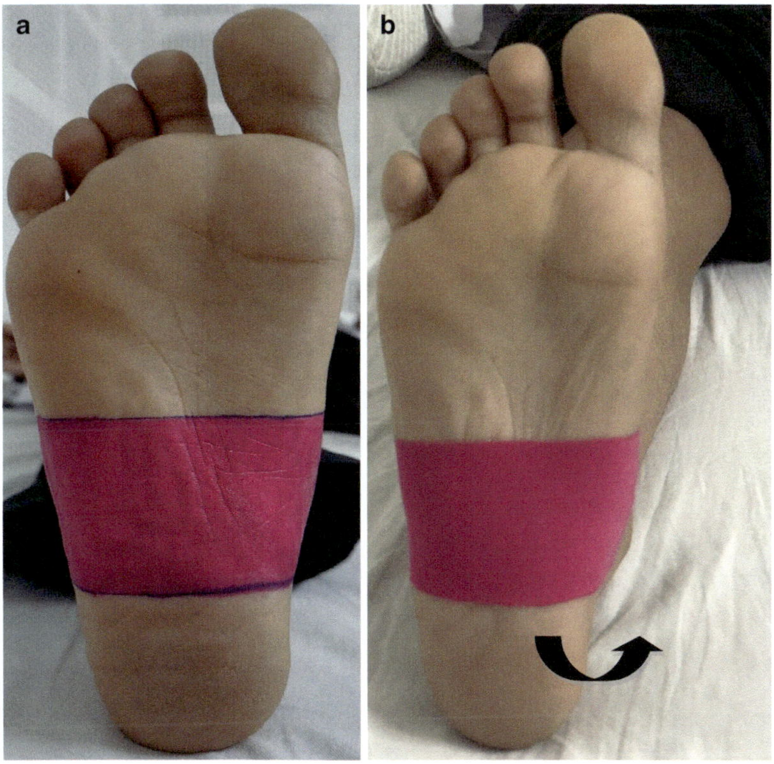

Fig. 7.15 (**a**) Marking of Transverse arch (**b**) NMT for Transverse arch

7.13 NMT for Tibialis Anterior

Patient position—supine with lower limbs in neutral position at hip, knee, and ankle.

Therapist position—standing by the side of the patient.

Procedure: The tape will be applied from the origin to the insertion of the tibialis anterior muscle without applying any tension. The tape extended from the upper two-thirds of the lateral surface of the tibia to the dorsum of the foot, encircling the first cuneiform and first metatarsal bone. Refer Fig. 7.16.

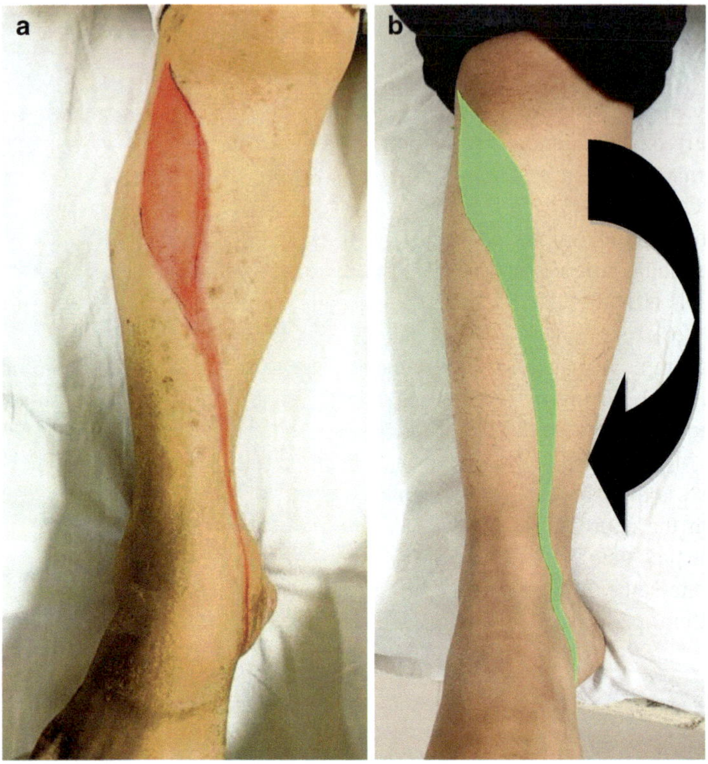

Fig. 7.16 (**a**) Marking for Tibialis Anterior muscle (**b**) NMT for Tibialis Anterior muscle

7.14 NMT for Tibialis Posterior

Patient position—prone with lower limbs in neutral position at hip, knee, and ankle.

Therapist position—standing by the side of the patient.

Procedure: Application of tape from the origin to the insertion of the posterior tibialis muscle without any stretch. This strip originated along the inner posterior borders of the tibia and fibula, extending over the muscle to reach around the medial malleolus. Refer Fig. 7.17.

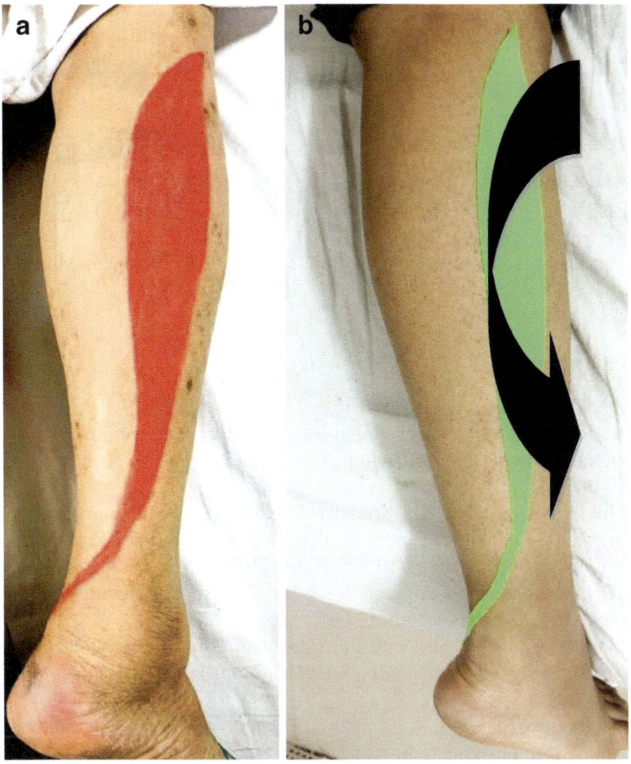

Fig. 7.17 (**a**) marking for tibialis posterior muscle (**b**) NMT for tibialis posterior muscle

7.15 NMT for Peroneus Longus

Patient position—prone with lower limbs in neutral position at hip, knee, and ankle.

Therapist position—standing by the side of the patient.

Procedure: The tape will be applied from the origin to the insertion of the peroneus longus muscle without any tension. This tape originated at the head of the fibula, traversed over the lateral malleolus, and extended beneath the plantar surface of the foot, concluding around the base of the first metatarsal. Refer Fig. 7.18.

In conclusion, it is evident that targeting peripheral nerves through various methods has been effective in alleviating sensorimotor complications associated with DPN. Techniques such as neural massage, neural mobilization, and neuromuscular taping show promise as treatments for DPN.

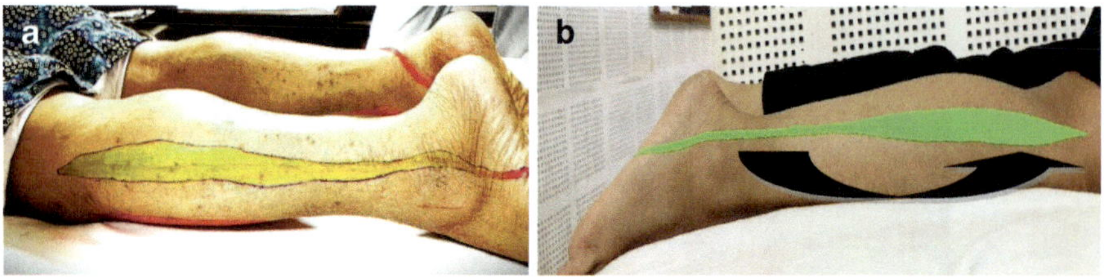

Fig. 7.18 (**a**) marking for Peroneus Longus muscle (**b**) NMT for Peroneus Muscle

References

1. Zilliox LA, Russell JW. Physical activity and dietary interventions in diabetic neuropathy: a systematic review. Clin Auton Res. 2019;29(4):443–55. https://doi.org/10.1007/s10286-019-00607-x.
2. Baum P, Toyka KV, Blüher M, Kosacka J, Nowicki M. Inflammatory mechanisms in the pathophysiology of diabetic peripheral neuropathy (DN)-new aspects. Int J Mol Sci. 2021;22(19):10835. https://doi.org/10.3390/ijms221910835.
3. Obrosova IG. Diabetes and the peripheral nerve. Biochim Biophys Acta. 2009;1792(10):931–40. https://doi.org/10.1016/j.bbadis.2008.11.005.
4. Frank T, Nawroth P, Kuner R. Structure-function relationships in peripheral nerve contributions to diabetic peripheral neuropathy. Pain. 2019;160(Suppl 1):S29–36. https://doi.org/10.1097/j.pain.0000000000001530.
5. Kluding PM, Pasnoor M, Singh R, Jernigan S, Farmer K, Rucker J, et al. The effect of exercise on neuropathic symptoms, nerve function, and cutaneous innervation in people with diabetic peripheral neuropathy. J Diabetes Complicat. 2012;26(5):424–9. https://doi.org/10.1016/j.jdiacomp.2012.05.007.
6. Zhu GC, Tsai KL, Chen YW, Hung CH. Neural mobilization attenuates mechanical allodynia and decreases proinflammatory cytokine concentrations in rats with painful diabetic neuropathy. Phys Ther. 2018;98(4):214–22. https://doi.org/10.1093/ptj/pzx124.
7. Callaghan BC, Cheng HT, Stables CL, Smith AL, Feldman EL. Diabetic neuropathy: clinical manifestations and current treatments. Lancet Neurol. 2012;11(6):521–34. https://doi.org/10.1016/S1474-4422(12)70065-0.
8. Galiero R, Caturano A, Vetrano E, Beccia D, Brin C, Alfano M, et al. Peripheral neuropathy in diabetes mellitus: pathogenetic mechanisms and diagnostic options. Int J Mol Sci. 2023;24(4):3554. https://doi.org/10.3390/ijms24043554.
9. Pop-Busui R, Boulton AJ, Feldman EL, Bril V, Freeman R, Malik RA, et al. Diabetic neuropathy: a position statement by the American Diabetes Association. Diabetes Care. 2017;40(1):136–54. https://doi.org/10.2337/dc16-2042.
10. Balducci S, Iacobellis G, Parisi L, Di Biase N, Calandriello E, Leonetti F, et al. Exercise training can modify the natural history of diabetic peripheral neuropathy. J Diabetes Complicat. 2006;20(4):216–23. https://doi.org/10.1016/j.jdiacomp.2005.07.005.
11. Said G. Diabetic neuropathy—a review. Nat Clin Pract Neurol. 2007;3(6):331–40. https://doi.org/10.1038/ncpneuro0504.
12. Juster-Switlyk K, Smith AG. Updates in diabetic peripheral neuropathy. F1000Res. 2016;5:F1000 Faculty Rev-738. https://doi.org/10.12688/f1000research.7898.1.
13. Breig A, Marions O. BIOMECHANICS OF THE LUMBOSACRAL NERVE ROOTS. Acta Radiol Diagn (Stockh). 1963;1:1141–60. https://doi.org/10.1177/028418516300100603.

14. Coppieters MW, Butler DS. Do 'sliders' slide and 'tensioners' tension? An analysis of neurodynamic techniques and considerations regarding their application. Man Ther. 2008;13(3):213–21. https://doi.org/10.1016/j.math.2006.12.008.
15. Butler D. Mobilisation of the nervous system. Melbourne: Churchill Livingstone; 1991.
16. Shacklock M. Neurodynamics. Physiotherapy. 1995;81(1):9–16. https://doi.org/10.1016/S0031-9406(05)67024-1.
17. Butler D, Gifford L. The concept of adverse mechanical tension in the nervous system. Part 1: testing for 'dural tension'. Physiotherapy. 1989a;75:622–9. https://doi.org/10.1016/S0031-9406(10)62374-7.
18. Butler D, Gifford L. The concept of adverse mechanical tension in the nervous system. Part 2: Examination and treatment. Physiotherapy. 1989;75:629–36. https://doi.org/10.1016/S0031-9406(10)62374-7.
19. Lima ÊM, Santana HHS, Medrado AP, Martinez AMB, Baptista AF. Neurodynamic mobilization reduces intraneural fibrosis after sciatic crush lesion in rats. Braz J Med Human Health. 2017;5(2):54–62. https://doi.org/10.17267/2317-3386bjmhh.v5i2.1303.
20. Castilho J, Ferreira LAB, Pereira WM, Neto HP, Morelli JGDS, Brandalize D, et al. Analysis of electromyographic activity in spastic biceps brachii muscle following neural mobilization. J Bodyw Mov Ther. 2012;16(3):364–8. https://doi.org/10.1016/j.jbmt.2011.12.003.
21. Ellis RF, Hing WA. Neural mobilization: a systematic review of randomized controlled trials with an analysis of therapeutic efficacy. J Man Manip Ther. 2008;16(1):8–22. https://doi.org/10.1179/106698108790818594.
22. Sharma R, Saxena A, Samuel A. A mixed-method study to explore individuals with stroke experiences of median nerve mobilization on spasticity and improving upper limb strength. Int J Stroke. 2023;18(S):255. https://doi.org/10.1177/17474930231192010.
23. Villafañe JH. Botulinum toxin type A combined with neurodynamic mobilization for lower limb spasticity: a case report. J Chiropr Med. 2013;12(1):39–44. https://doi.org/10.1016/j.jcm.2013.01.001.
24. Villafañe JH, Silva GB, Chiarotto A, Ragusa OL. Botulinum toxin type A combined with neurodynamic mobilization for upper limb spasticity after stroke: a case report. J Chiropr Med. 2012;11(3):186–91. https://doi.org/10.1016/j.jcm.2012.05.009.
25. Cha HK, Cho HS, Choi JD. Effects of the nerve mobilization technique on lower limb function in patients with poststroke hemiparesis. J Phys Ther Sci. 2014;26(7):981–3. https://doi.org/10.1589/jpts.26.981.
26. Saxena A, Sehgal S, Jangra MK. Effectiveness of neurodynamic mobilization versus conventional therapy on spasticity reduction and upper limb function in tetraplegic patients. Asian Spine J. 2021;15(4):498–503. https://doi.org/10.31616/asj.2020.0146.
27. Villafañe JH, Pillastrini P, Borboni A. Manual therapy and neurodynamic mobilization in a patient with peroneal nerve paralysis: a case report. J Chiropr Med. 2013;12(3):176–81. https://doi.org/10.1016/j.jcm.2013.10.007.
28. Kumar PS, Adhikari P, Jeganathan PS, D'Souza SC. Immediate effects of nerve sliders and nerve massage on vibration and thermal perception thresholds in patients with painful diabetic peripheral neuropathy- a pilot randomized clinical trial (UTRN 103229513-050820102510203). Physiother Occup Ther J. 2010;3(3):5–19.
29. Nee RJ, Butler D. Management of peripheral neuropathic pain: integrating neurobiology, neurodynamics, and clinical evidence. Phys Ther Sport. 2006;7(1):36–49. https://doi.org/10.1016/j.ptsp.2005.10.002.
30. Chen YW, Hsieh PL, Chen YC, Hung CH, Cheng JT. Physical exercise induces excess hsp72 expression and delays the development of hyperalgesia and allodynia in painful diabetic neuropathy rats. Anesth Analg. 2013;116(2):482–90. https://doi.org/10.1213/ANE.0b013e318274e4a0.

31. Zhu GC, Chen YW, Tsai KL, Wang JJ, Hung CH, Schmid AB. Effects of neural mobilization on sensory dysfunction and peripheral nerve degeneration in rats with painful diabetic neuropathy. Phys Ther. 2022;102(10):pzac104. https://doi.org/10.1093/ptj/pzac104.
32. da Silva JT, Santos FM, Giardini AC, Martins Dde O, de Oliveira ME, Ciena AP, et al. Neural mobilization promotes nerve regeneration by nerve growth factor and myelin protein zero increased after sciatic nerve injury. Growth Factors. 2015;33(1):8–13. https://doi.org/10.3109/08977194.2014.953630.
33. Goyal M, Esht V, Mittal A. A study protocol on nerve mobilization induced diffusion tensor imaging values in posterior tibial nerve in healthy controls and in patients with diabetic neuropathy-multigroup pretest posttest design. Contemp Clin Trials Commun. 2019;16:100451. https://doi.org/10.1016/j.conctc.2019.100451.
34. Kumar PS, Adhikari P, Jeganathan PS. Immediate effects of longitudinal vs. transverse tibial nerve massage on vibration perception thresholds and thermal perception thresholds in asymptomatic subjects: a pilot randomized clinical trial (UTRN 014427448-2101200878203). Occup Ther J. 2010;3(1):13–23.
35. Goyal M, Mittal A, Samuel AJ. Effect of massage, passive neural mobilization and transcutaneous electrical nerve stimulation on magnetic resonance diffusion tensor imaging (MR-DTI) of the tibial nerve in a patient with type 2 diabetes mellitus induced neuropathy: a case report. Physiother Theory Pract. 2022;38(13):3273–82. https://doi.org/10.1080/09593985.2021.1994070.
36. Alshimy AM, Ibrahim SM, Osama L, Metwally HM. Effect of neurodynamic mobilization techniques in patients with diabetic neuropathy. Human Movement. 2023;24(3):115–20. https://doi.org/10.5114/hm.2023.121656.
37. Moksha J, Medha D, Swati M. Effectiveness of sliders vs tensioners on pain and disability in nonspecific low back pain with associated lower limb symptoms: a pretest posttest experimental study. IJHSR. 2019;9(9):46–52.
38. Lim JY, Lee IW, Kim KD. Immediate effects of neural slider and neural tensioner on forward bending in subjects with hamstring tightness. J Musculoskelet Sci Technol. 2021;5(1):6–13.
39. Morsi HI, El Nahass BG, Ibrahim MM. Effects of slider, tensioner neurodynamic mobilization techniques and stretching exercises in treatment of chronic discogenic sciatica: a comparative study. J Muscuoskelet Res. 2022; https://doi.org/10.21203/rs.3.rs-1572951/v1.
40. Papacharalambous C, Savva C, Karagiannis C, Giannakou K. The effectiveness of slider and tensioner neural mobilization techniques in the management of upper quadrant pain: a systematic review of randomized controlled trials. J Bodyw Mov Ther. 2022;31:102–12. https://doi.org/10.1016/j.jbmt.2022.03.002.
41. Brown CL, Gilbert KK, Brismee JM, Sizer PS, Roger James C, Smith MP. The effects of neurodynamic mobilization on fluid dispersion within the tibial nerve at the ankle: an unembalmed cadaveric study. J Man Manip Ther. 2011;19(1):26–34. https://doi.org/10.1179/2042618610Y.0000000003.
42. Goyat M, Saxena A, Goyal M. Study Protocol titled as "Effectiveness of neural mobilization in improving the ankle ROM and plantar pressure distribution in patients with diabetic peripheral neuropathy: a single group, pre post, quasi experimental study protocol". J Diabetes Metab Disord. 2022;21(2):2035–41. https://doi.org/10.1007/s40200-022-01106-z.
43. Shacklock MO. Clinical neurodynamics: a new system of musculoskeletal treatment. Edinburgh, New York: Elsevier Butterworth-Heinemann; 2005.
44. Kristianto H, Waluyo A, Gayatri D, Yunir E, Blow D. Neuromuscular taping treatment of diabetic foot: a concept analysis. Clin Ter. 2021;172(3):231–5.
45. Kristianto H, Waluyo A, Yunir E, Gayatri D, Blow D. Neuromuscular taping application opportunities in nursing: a literature review. Central EuroJ Nurs Midwifery. 2020;11(3):143–51.
46. Susanti I, Arofiati F. The effectiveness of Neuromuscular Taping (NMT) and foot exercise in improving microsirculations in diabetes mellitus patients. Jurnal Aisyah: Jurnal Ilmu Kesehatan. 2022;7(S2):71–8.

47. Berlingeri C, Camerota F, Celletti C, Turolla A, Peraro A, Blow D, et al. Possible applications of Neuromuscular Taping in pain reduction in Multiple Sclerosis subject: a preliminary report. Senses Sci. 2016;3(4):303–7.
48. Camerota F, Galli M, Cimolin V, Celletti C, Ancillao A, Blow D, et al. Neuromuscular taping for the upper limb in cerebral palsy: a case study in a patient with hemiplegia. Dev Neurorehabil. 2014;17(6):384–7.
49. Muchsin AH, Blow D, Goysal Y, Tammasse J, Bahar A, Wuysang AD, et al. Neuromuscular taping decompression technique in diabetic painful distal symmetrical polyneuropathy: the impact on pain intensity in a randomised trial. Res Square. 2023; https://doi.org/10.21203/rs.3.rs-2509764/v1.
50. Thakur K, Goyal M. Effectiveness of neuromuscular taping on balance, proprioception, pain, and nerve conduction parameters in patients with diabetic peripheral neuropathy: a two-group pretest-posttest randomized sham-controlled trial study protocol. J Diabetes Metab Disord. 2023;22(2):1793–800. https://doi.org/10.1007/s40200-023-01275-5.

Chapter 8
Role of Orthotics in the Management of Diabetic Peripheral Neuropathy

Urvi and Shweta Sharma

Contents

8.1 Introduction

Diabetes mellitus has become a persistent public health emergency worldwide in the twenty-first century. Diabetes currently affects 115 million people in China [1], 73 million in India [2], and 30 million in the USA [3]. As the cases of diabetes mellitus are at an all-time high worldwide, understandably its complications have become another menace health providers have to deal with globally. Out of these innumerable complications, a group of clinical syndromes, generally referred to as

Urvi
Physiotherapy, SGT University, Gurugram, Haryana, India

S. Sharma (✉)
MM Institute of Physiotherapy & Rehabilitation, Maharishi Markandeshwar (Deemed to be University), Ambala, Haryana, India
e-mail: Shweta.sharma@mmumullana.org

© The Author(s), under exclusive license to Springer Nature Singapore Pte Ltd. 2024

M. Goyal, K. Goyal (eds.), *Rehabilitation in Diabetic Peripheral Neuropathy*, https://doi.org/10.1007/978-981-97-9290-0_8

different forms of neuropathy are most prevalent, caused by damage to peripheral and autonomic nervous systems [4]. Among these, diabetic peripheral neuropathy is quite rampant and debilitating complication, causing severe distress to diabetic patients worldwide [5]. Defined as nerve damage of the extremities caused due to chronically high levels of blood glucose, diabetic peripheral neuropathy leads to significant complications and decrease in quality of life [6]. Along with life hampering setbacks, diabetic peripheral neuropathy has significant effect on healthcare economics as well [7]. 20% of all diabetic hospital visits in the USA are attributed to neuropathic foot issues, which are projected to cost the UK £252 million yearly [8]. The cost of treating a neuropathic ulcer varies based on its location and severity, ranging from US$7000 to US$28,000. If an amputation is required, the cost might reach $50,000 or $60,000 [9, 10].

Orthotic therapies are essential for controlling the effects of diabetic peripheral neuropathy, especially when it comes to avoiding difficulties and maintaining mobility. Orthotics provide a non-invasive method of relieving pressure, redistributing forces, and improving equilibrium in the lower limbs [11]. The foot is a typical location of difficulties in diabetic peripheral neuropathy. Orthotics play a vital role in preventing foot ulcers, lowering the risk of infections, and eventually avoiding the need for more intrusive operations like amputations by offering support and protection. Orthotic therapies are important in the larger context of healthcare resource allocation and economics. Over time, orthotics can save a significant amount of money by averting problems like amputations and foot ulcers.

This chapter aims to give a thorough examination of the dynamic interaction that exists between diabetic peripheral neuropathy and orthotic therapies. This chapter seeks to clarify the ways in which orthotics aid in the treatment and avoidance of diabetic peripheral neuropathy-related issues by synthesizing recent research findings, clinical experiences, and technical developments. In order to help healthcare practitioners, researchers, and educators better understand DPN and its management through orthotic interventions, this chapter aims to close the gap between theoretical understanding and actual implementation.

8.2 Understanding DPN

Diabetic peripheral neuropathy (DPN) is a crippling kind of nerve injury that mostly affects the peripheral nerves in people with diabetes [6]. These peripheral nerves are crucial for the transmission of messages from the central nervous system to different body areas, which control vital processes including sensation and movement [12]. This is a complex neurological condition where long-term exposure to high blood glucose sets off a series of events that eventually cause severe peripheral nerve damage and dysfunction.

Several research works highlight the complex connection between hyperglycemia and diabetic peripheral neuropathy development (Fig. 8.1). This type of neuropathy affects almost 50% of people with diabetes in their lifetime, demonstrating

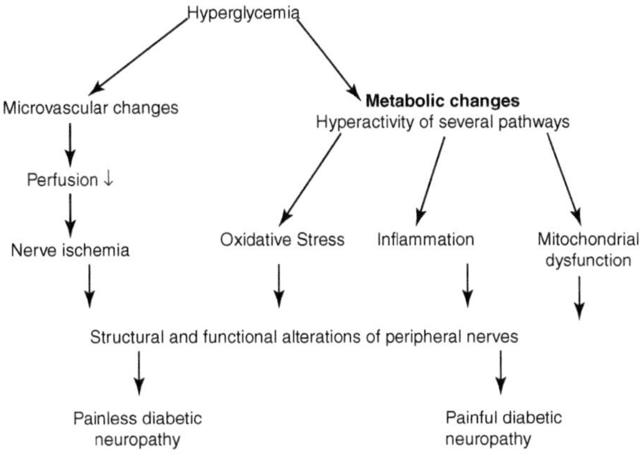

Fig. 8.1 Pathophysiology of diabetic peripheral neuropathy [13]

Table 8.1 Clinical presentation [14]

Numbness in hands/feet/both: Stocking glove distribution
Tingling/burning sensation in feet
Pain in hands/feet
Dry/cracked feet
Foot drop or tripping

the complication's broad prevalence. Moreover, poor glycemic management, the length of diabetes, and other risk factors including obesity and smoking all increase the chance of acquiring DPN. This emphasizes how critical it is to have a thorough grasp of DPN in order to improve management techniques, diagnostic precision, and preventative measures.

Diabetic peripheral neuropathy is a notable and often occurring consequence of diabetes that significantly impairs the quality of life for those who experience it. The impact of diabetic peripheral neuropathy on foot health is pretty alarming due to which healthcare providers are concerned worldwide (Table 8.1). The reason for this impact is considered to be the vulnerable nature of feet to sensory and blood flow deficits. As chronic diabetic peripheral neuropathy can lead to loss of pain perception, leading to negligence in foot related care and injuries, patients become vulnerable to a condition called diabetic foot ulcers (DFU). Such serious effects of diabetic peripheral neuropathy (DPN) on foot health are highlighted by the fact that those with diabetes have a 12-fold increased risk of lower limb amputation when compared to those without the disease [15].

Also, development of foot deformities pertaining to diabetic peripheral neuropathy is another menace patients and healthcare providers have to deal with globally. Prevalence of deformities such as foot drop, Charcot's arthropathy are rampant among such patients which further accentuates occurrence of various mentioned complications leading to poor quality of life [16]. Therefore, vigilant foot care in diabetes and diabetic peripheral neuropathy must be considered of utmost importance when dealing with cases of diabetes of various types.

8.3 Role of Orthotics

Orthoses are orthopedic appliances that help to improve or prevent deformity and provide support, alignment, and correction for deformities [17]. When discussing diabetic foot care, orthotics refer to externally applied tools that are intended to support, adjust, or change the function of the musculoskeletal and neuromuscular systems. Healthcare providers have been using foot orthoses for more than 150 years to treat musculoskeletal disorders, prevent injuries, and improve lower limb biomechanics [18]. These gadgets fit into shoes and can be manufactured to order or prefabricated. The goals of orthotics are to improve general foot function, reduce discomfort, and treat abnormalities. In medical literature, following objectives for utilization of foot orthosis are identified (Table 8.2).

8.3.1 Classification of Orthotics

8.3.1.1 Custom Orthotics

These custom-made gadgets are constructed from an intricate foot imprint and are intended to treat specific biomechanical foot problems. Patients with diabetic peripheral neuropathy, who require accommodations for specific pressure sites, have distinct foot deformities, or have major structural variations in their feet can benefit most from custom orthotics [20].

8.3.1.2 Over-the-Counter Orthotics (OTC)

These are mass manufactured inserts providing stability and padding for a variety of foot sizes and shapes and are freely available without a prescription. When awaiting bespoke orthotics, OTC orthotics might offer DPN sufferers with minor symptoms some early alleviation or an interim solution [11].

Table 8.2 Objectives for utilization of foot orthoses [19]

1. Shock attenuation and absorption
2. Cushioning to tender areas of foot
3. Relieve areas of abnormally increased plantar pressure
4. Support and protection of healed fracture site
5. Minimization of shear forces
6. Correction, support and stabilization of flexible deformities
7. Restriction of motion in painful joints
8. Accommodate for rigid deformities.

8.3.1.3 Soft Orthotics

These orthotics, which are made of cushioned materials, are intended to improve balance, reduce pressure on painful or bothersome foot regions, and absorb shock [21]. They assist transmit pressure uniformly over the foot, making them suitable for DPN patients with extreme foot deformities, hypersensitive feet, or those at high risk of ulceration.

8.3.1.4 Rigid Orthotics

Rigid orthotics are made of stiff materials (Table 8.3) and are intended to manage function by limiting aberrant foot mobility. Due to the degree of hardness, they are less frequently utilized in DPN, but for individuals who have certain alignment problems that lead to foot discomfort or instability, they could be helpful [16].

8.3.1.5 Semi-Rigid Orthotics

These orthotics, which combine hard and soft materials (Table 8.3), provide skeletal assistance and padding to assist improvement in foot balance on surfaces that are uneven. For DPN patients who are active and need both comfort and correction, such those who play sports, semi-rigid orthotics might be helpful [16].

8.3.2 *Fabrication Process (Fig. 8.2)*

Fabrication process of orthosis includes several crucial steps each of which must be followed with discipline:

8.3.2.1 Comprehensive Foot Assessment

The first and foremost step of fabrication process is comprehensive and thorough foot assessment. It may include complete physical examination including closely observing the surface of foot, biomechanical assessment including deformity analysis if present and assessment of peripheral artery disease (PAD).

Table 8.3 Common materials used in orthotics [16]

1. Polyethylene and polypropylene	Rigid materials ideal for providing support.
2. Carbon fiber	Provides strength and support without significant bulk. Thus, is ideal for active patients requiring minimal modifications.
3. Ethylene-vinyl acetate (EVA)	Cushioning material, ideal for sensitive areas of foot.
4. Leather	Added on the top-most layer for refinement and breathability.

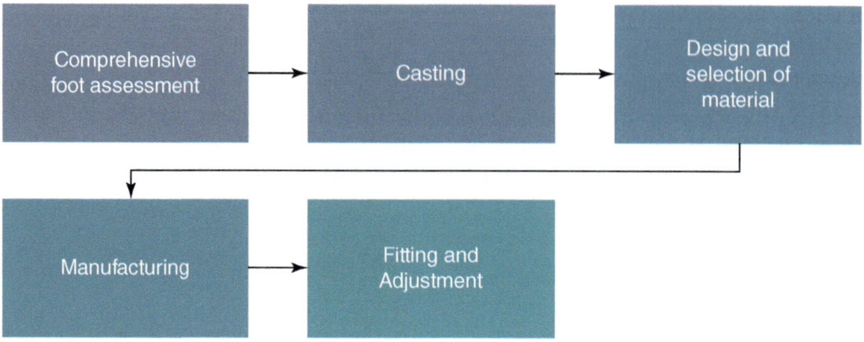

Fig. 8.2 Steps in manufacturing of orthotics

8.3.2.2 Casting

In next step, the foot is casted to produce an exact mold. There are several different methods, such as 3D scanning, foam box imprints, and plaster casting. The objective is to precisely record the foot's features in its most advantageous alignment.

8.3.2.3 Design and Selection of Material

The orthotic is developed based on the evaluation and casting done in first and second step. At this stage, the form, thickness, and materials for the orthotic—which should be customized based on the patient's unique foot problems, activity level, and footwear—are decided upon.

8.3.2.4 Manufacturing

After meticulously following the previous steps, the unique design of orthotic is made. This might entail a variety of methods, such as computer-aided manufacturing procedures that guarantee a high level of precision or handcrafting based on the mold.

8.3.2.5 Fitting and Adjustment

After the orthotics are made, the patient has them fitted to their appropriate footwear. Along with this, patient's comfort and efficacy are evaluated. To make sure everything fits and works well, adjustments can be made.

8.3.3 Overview of Types of Orthotics for DPN

8.3.3.1 Insoles/ Orthotic Inserts (Fig. 8.3)

A form of assistive device, insole/orthotic inserts is prescribed to correct biomechanical asymmetries and pain [22]. By impairing the peripheral nerve system and decreasing sensory inputs, peripheral neuropathy progressively causes postural instability [23–25]. In other words, because the somatosensory, visual, and vestibular systems are involved in managing balance, diabetic neuropathy is linked to an increased risk of falling [26]. Balance is significantly improved by using textured insoles. The senses, particularly proprioception and tactile senses, appear to be most affected by the firm textured insole. Patients with diabetic neuropathy see an enhancement in balance as a result of stimulation of the deep receptors in their soles [27]. Consequently, it is possible to prescribe the use of hard-textured insoles as a non-invasive, inexpensive, and simple solution.

8.3.3.2 Ankle-Foot Orthoses (Fig. 8.4)

Diabetic peripheral neuropathy is known to affect strength of dorsiflexor muscles resulting in foot drop. Increased hip and knee flexion are compensatory measures that are triggered by foot drop, which limits gait capacity and prevents tripping [28]. Foot drop might only be noticeable when muscles fatigue, and it could also be linked to evertor weakness, which lowers medial-lateral stability.

Conservative measures such as prescribing ankle-foot orthoses (AFOs) are frequently used to lessen foot drop and enhance gait [29]. Their purpose is to limit plantar flexion through the swing phase of gait, therefore compensating for the absence of active dorsiflexion [29]. While AFOs don't normalize gait patterns, they

Fig. 8.3 Orthotic inserts/ insoles

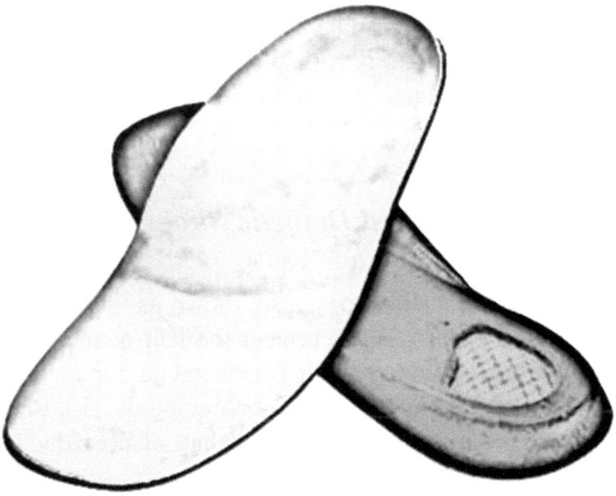

Fig. 8.4 Ankle-foot orthosis

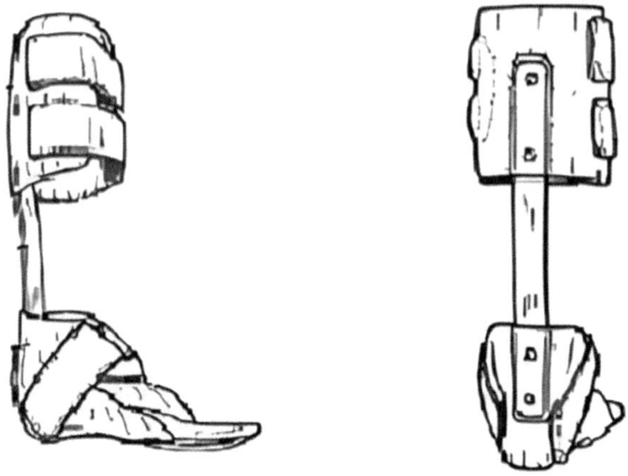

do decrease kinematic and kinetic abnormalities, which lowers the risk of falls and compensatory techniques while also increasing gait capacity, which may make participation easier [30, 31].

8.3.3.3 Footwear Modifications (Fig. 8.5)

Practically made to protect the feet of diabetics, particularly those with diabetic peripheral neuropathy (DPN), specialized diabetic shoes, sometimes referred to as extra-depth shoes or therapeutic shoes are often prescribed. The danger of foot injuries, comfort, and the avoidance of problems like ulcers, calluses, and sores that can develop from the disease's effect on foot health are all made possible by these shoes, which are essential for diabetic foot care [32]. Some of its key features [16] are as follows:

- Extra depth—to accommodate orthotic insoles and redirect pressure on foot.
- Smooth interior—to prevent abrasions and wear and tear on skin of foot.
- Rocker soles—promote natural gait by reducing pressure on ball of foot.
- Wide toe box—to prevent blisters and ulcers on toes.
- Firm heel counters—to control motion of foot and prevent disbalance and falls.

8.3.4 Specialized Diabetic Shoes

Specialized diabetic shoes, also known as therapeutic shoes or extra-depth shoes, are carefully designed to protect the feet of individuals with diabetes, especially those suffering from diabetic peripheral neuropathy (DPN). These shoes play a crucial role in diabetic foot care by reducing the risk of foot injuries, promoting comfort, and preventing complications that can arise due to the disease's impact on foot health, such as ulcers, calluses, and sores.

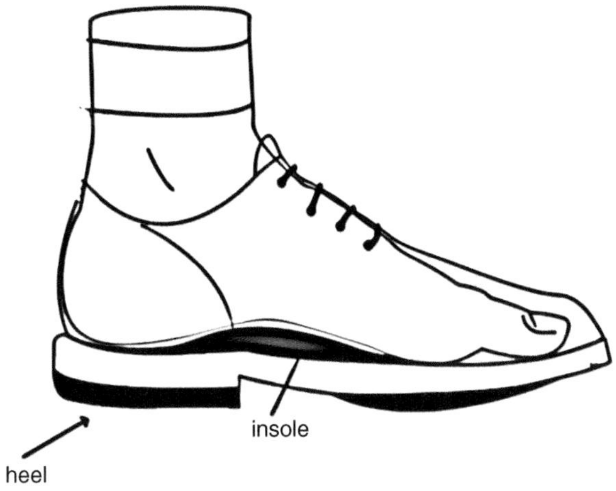

Fig. 8.5 Modified footwear

8.3.4.1 Key Features of Specialized Diabetic Shoes

8.3.4.1.1 Extra Depth

To accommodate custom orthotics or insoles, diabetic shoes are deeper than standard footwear. This extra space helps in pressure redistribution across the foot, minimizing the risk of pressure sores.

8.3.4.1.2 Non-Binding Uppers

The upper part of the shoe is soft and made from flexible materials that do not constrict or bind the foot, reducing pressure points and improving comfort for sensitive areas.

8.3.4.1.3 Seamless Interior

A smooth, seamless interior is critical to prevent irritation and abrasions, especially in areas where the skin is vulnerable to breaking down.

8.3.4.1.4 Wide Toe Box

A spacious toe box gives toes ample room, reducing pressure on the toes and preventing blisters, calluses, and ulcers.

8.3.4.1.5 Rocker Soles

Designed to reduce pressure in the ball-of-the-foot area, rocker soles help in promoting a natural gait, thus aiding mobility and reducing strain.

8.3.4.1.6 Firm Heel Counters

Provide stability and support, helping in controlling the motion of the foot to reduce the risk of injuries.

8.3.5 Clinical Considerations for Orthotic Prescription in DPN

8.3.5.1 Assessment of Neuropathy Severity

A thorough assessment of severity of neuropathy must be done by clinicians using universally accepted and validated assessment tools. Orthotic interventions must be tailored based on the degree of sensory and motor disabilities and deformities. Michigan Neuropathy Screening Instrument (MNSI) and Neuropathy Disability Score (NDS) are examples of globally accepted and used tools for screening neuropathies [33, 34].

8.3.5.2 Assessment of Peripheral Artery Disease (PAD)

Assessment of foot blood regulation is also an important aspect that most clinicians tend to ignore while prescribing foot orthotics. Any underlying PAD can be worsened if improper orthotics are prescribed without considering this factor. Assessment of pedal pulses and ankle-brachial index test are some of the ways through which peripheral artery disease presence can be assessed [35].

8.3.5.3 Pressure Redistribution

The type of orthotic to be prescribed must be carefully selected and must accommodate proper pressure redistribution to prevent skin abrasions, rashes, and ulcers which can be detrimental in terms of patient's quality of life and prognosis of the disease [36].

8.3.5.4 Footwear Recommendations

Patients must be properly advised to wear appropriate footwears along with the prescribed orthotic at all times to prevent friction injuries and prolonging the life of the assistive device [37].

8.3.5.5 Proper Wearing and Removing Techniques

Patients must be thoroughly taught the proper technique of wearing and removing the prescribed orthotic. Improperly worn orthotic can potentially alter the biomechanics of target joint in a detrimental way and can lead to increased complications. Removal technique must also be emphasized so as to prevent damage to the orthotic device and in turn maintain its longevity [37].

8.3.5.6 Body Weight

Patient's body weight must also be taken into account while prescribing orthoses. High body weight can increase contact pressure between surface of foot and sole of orthosis leading to foot ulcers and contact injuries. To tackle this, appropriate insoles should be added in the orthotic with proper cushioning [38].

8.3.6 Patient Education

Patient education is an important and understated aspect of orthotic management. Some of its salient features are as follows:

8.3.6.1 Foot Care and Inspection

Patients must be educated on daily self-feet inspections which include regularly checking for blisters, cuts, redness or swelling. Any abnormalities should be immediately reported to the primary health provider [39].

8.3.6.2 Foot Hygiene

Maintenance of proper foot hygiene should be emphasized which includes proper washing and drying, especially the areas between toes. Thorough moisturization of foot must be done to prevent cracked and dry skin.[40]

8.3.6.3 Protection of Feet

Feet must be protected at all cost from extreme temperatures, sharp objects, and other potential sources of injury. Appropriate usage of footwear must be encouraged and walking barefoot, especially outside home-setting must be totally discouraged [40].

8.3.6.4 Regular Check-Ups

Timely follow-up check-ups must be done with healthcare professionals for ensuring regular medical monitoring of foot health so that any concerns can be timely addressed [39].

8.4 Conclusion

This comprehensive exploration of role of orthotics in management of diabetic peripheral neuropathy (DPN) has revealed numerous new developments and breakthroughs in worldwide diabetic care. Adding orthotics to clinical practice is a great way to supplement conventional methods and medication-based therapies. Orthotics should be viewed by medical professionals as an essential part of a patient-centered, individualized treatment strategy for people with diabetic peripheral neuropathy. Given that DPN presentations are complex, orthotic prescriptions should be customized to the unique biomechanical and neuropathic profile of each patient. To guarantee the best possible results and make necessary adjustments to treatments, routine clinical follow-ups should incorporate regular monitoring and appraisal of orthotic efficacy.

Barriers including cost, accessibility, and patient education must also be addressed in order to successfully integrate orthotics into clinical practice. Efforts aimed at reducing the cost and increasing the availability of orthotic therapies, in conjunction with extensive patient education initiatives, have the potential to augment their implementation across various healthcare environments.

A multidisciplinary approach that goes beyond conventional medical therapies is necessary due to the intricacy of diabetic peripheral neuropathy. To effectively handle the many aspects of DPN, orthotists, podiatrists, endocrinologists, physiotherapists, and other healthcare practitioners must work together fluidly. A unified and patient-focused strategy may be ensured through joint decision-making procedures, which are aided by frequent case conferences and collaborative care models. It is also crucial to include patient education programs that stress the value of orthotic therapies and self-care routines. Giving people with diabetic peripheral neuropathy the tools they need to actively engage in their care, improves treatment compliance and gives them a sense of independence in managing their illness.

Using orthotics as a useful tool in their toolbox, medical professionals may customize therapies to meet the specific needs of each patient and participate in continuous multidisciplinary teamwork. By doing this, medical professionals may improve the general standard of care provided to people with DPN, which will ultimately lead to better functional results and a higher standard of living.

Future developments in orthotics research and innovation, along with a dedication to interdisciplinary cooperation, will open the door for completer and more successful DPN management strategies. One major step toward a patient-centered, integrated perspective in the treatment of diabetic peripheral neuropathy patients is the normal clinical practice of using orthotics.

References

1. Wang L, Gao P, Zhang M, Huang Z, Zhang D, Deng Q, et al. Prevalence and ethnic pattern of diabetes and prediabetes in China in 2013. JAMA. 2017;317(24):2515–23. https://doi.org/10.1001/jama.2017.7596.
2. Anjana RM, Deepa M, Pradeepa R, Mahanta J, Narain K, Das HK, et al. Prevalence of diabetes and prediabetes in 15 states of India: results from the ICMR-INDIAB population-based cross-sectional study. Lancet Diabetes Endocrinol. 2017;5(8):585–96. https://doi.org/10.1016/S2213-8587(17)30174-2.
3. Henderson CE, Nezam H, Castillo KM. Centers for disease control and prevention-recognized diabetes prevention program after gestational diabetes mellitus. AJOG Glob Rep. 2022;3(1):100150. https://doi.org/10.1016/j.xagr.2022.100150.
4. Feldman EL, Callaghan BC, Pop-Busui R, Zochodne DW, Wright DE, Bennett DL, Bril V, Russell JW, Viswanathan V. Diabetic neuropathy. Nat Rev Dis Primers. 2019;5(1):42. https://doi.org/10.1038/s41572-019-0097-9.
5. Pfannkuche A, Alhajjar A, Ming A, Walter I, Piehler C, Mertens PR. Prevalence and risk factors of diabetic peripheral neuropathy in a diabetics' cohort: register initiative "diabetes and nerves". Endocr Metabol Sci. 2020;1(1–2):100053. https://doi.org/10.1016/j.endmts.2020.100053.
6. Bodman MA, Dreyer MA, Varacallo M. Diabetic peripheral neuropathy. 2024 Feb 25. In: StatPearls [Internet]. Treasure Island (FL): StatPearls Publishing; 2024 Jan–. PMID: 28723038.
7. Robinson C, Major MJ, Kuffel C, Hines K, Cole P. Orthotic management of the neuropathic foot: an interdisciplinary care perspective. Prosthetics Orthot Int. 2015;39(1):73–81. https://doi.org/10.1177/0309364614545422.
8. Paton J, Bruce G, Jones R, et al. Effectiveness of insoles used for the prevention of ulceration in the neuropathic diabetic foot: a systematic review. J Diabetes Complicat. 2011;25:52–62.
9. Cavanagh PR, Lipsky BA, Bradbury AW, et al. Treatment for diabetic foot ulcers. Lancet. 2005;366:1725–35.
10. McKea S, Ross JJ, Dressler DD, et al. Principles and practice of hospital medicine. 1st ed. New York: McGraw-Hill Medical; 2012. p. 2310.
11. Mohaddis M, Maqsood SA, Ago E, Singh S, Naim Z, Prasad S. Enhancing functional rehabilitation through orthotic interventions for foot and ankle conditions: a narrative review. Cureus. 2023;15(11):e49103. https://doi.org/10.7759/cureus.49103.
12. Wilkinson JL. Chapter 3—Peripheral nervous system, neuroanatomy for medical students. 2nd ed. Butterworth-Heinemann; 1992. p. 32–51.
13. Sloan G, Selvarajah D, Tesfaye S. Pathogenesis, diagnosis and clinical management of diabetic sensorimotor peripheral neuropathy. Nat Rev Endocrinol. 2021;17(7):400–20. https://doi.org/10.1038/s41574-021-00496-z.

14. Kartha C, Ramachandran S, Pillai RM, editors. Mechanisms of vascular defects in diabetes mellitus. Springer; 2017. p. 163.
15. Armstrong DG, Boulton AJM, Bus SA. Diabetic foot ulcers and their recurrence. N Engl J Med. 2017;376(24):2367–75. https://doi.org/10.1056/NEJMra1615439.
16. Chang MC, Choo YJ, Park IS, Park MW, Kim DH. Orthotic approach to prevention and management of diabetic foot: a narrative review. World J Diabetes. 2022;13(11):912–20. https://doi.org/10.4239/wjd.v13.i11.912.
17. Khan MN, Jacobs BC, Ashbaugh S. Considerations in footwear and orthotics. Prim Care. 2013;40(4):1001–12, x. https://doi.org/10.1016/j.pop.2013.08.013.
18. Werd MB, Knight E, Langer PR. Athletic footwear and orthoses in sports medicine. Berlin: Springer Nature; 2010.
19. Janisse DJ. A scientific approach to insole design for the diabetic foot. Foot. 1993;3(3):105–8.
20. Barbara AM, Horton J. Custom-made foot orthotics for people with lower limb conditions: CADTH health technology review [internet]. Ottawa (ON): Canadian Agency for Drugs and Technologies in Health; 2022 Available from: https://www.ncbi.nlm.nih.gov/books/NBK595390/.
21. Peng HT, Liu LW, Chen CJ, Chen ZR. The soft prefabricated orthopedic insole decreases plantar pressure during uphill walking with heavy load carriage. Bioengineering (Basel). 2023;10(3):353. https://doi.org/10.3390/bioengineering10030353.
22. Menez C, L'Hermette M, Coquart J. Orthotic insoles improve gait symmetry and reduce immediate pain in subjects with mild leg length discrepancy. Front Sports Act Living. 2020;2:579152. https://doi.org/10.3389/fspor.2020.579152.
23. Guerrero CJV, Piraquive MAB, Saboyá ELS, et al. The diabetic foot: a review. Int J Collab Res Intern Med Public Health. 2020;12:972–7.
24. Khan KS, Andersen H. The impact of diabetic neuropathy on activities of daily living, postural balance and risk of falls-a systematic review. J Diabetes Sci Technol. 2022;16:289–94.
25. Asif M, Batool S. Association between diabetic neuropathy, fall risks and balance in diabetes type 2 patients. Rawal Med J. 2020;45(1):27–30.
26. Gioacchini FM, Albera R, Re M, et al. Hyperglycemia and diabetes mellitus are related to vestibular organs dysfunction: truth or suggestion? A literature review. Acta Diabetol. 2018;55:1201–7.
27. Alaee SJ, Barati K, Hajiaghaei B, Ghomian B, Moradi S, Poorpirali M. Immediate effect of textured insoles on the balance in patients with diabetic neuropathy. J Diabetes Investig. 2023;14(3):435–40. https://doi.org/10.1111/jdi.13950.
28. Don R, Serrao M, Vinci P, Ranavolo A, Cacchio A, Ioppolo F, et al. Foot drop and plantar flexion failure determine different gait strategies in Charcot-Marie-Tooth patients. Clin Biomech. 2007;22(8):905–16.
29. Menotti F, Laudani L, Damiani A, Orlando P, Macaluso A. Comparison of walking energy cost between an anterior and a posterior ankle-foot orthosis in people with foot drop. J Rehabil Med. 2014;46(8):768–72.
30. Ramdharry GM, Day BL, Reilly MM, Marsden JF. Foot drop splints improve proximal as well as distal leg control during gait in Charcot-Marie-Tooth Disease. Muscle Nerve. 2012;46(4):512–9.
31. Tyson SF, Sadeghi-Demneh E, Nester CJ. A systematic review and meta-analysis of the effect of an ankle-foot orthosis on gait biomechanics after stroke. Clin Rehabil. 2013;27(10):879–91.
32. Bus SA, Haspels R, Busch-Westbroek TE. Evaluation and optimization of therapeutic footwear for neuropathic diabetic foot patients using in-shoe plantar pressure analysis. Diabetes Care. 2011;34(7):1595–600. https://doi.org/10.2337/dc10-2206.
33. Herman WH, Pop-Busui R, Braffett BH, Martin CL, Cleary PA, Albers JW, Feldman EL, DCCT/EDIC Research Group. Use of the Michigan Neuropathy Screening Instrument as a measure of distal symmetrical peripheral neuropathy in Type 1 diabetes: results from the Diabetes Control and Complications Trial/Epidemiology of Diabetes Interventions and Complications. Diabet Med. 2012;29(7):937–44. https://doi.org/10.1111/j.1464-5491.2012.03644.

34. Yang Z, Chen R, Zhang Y, Huang Y, Hong T, Sun F, Ji L, Zhan S. Scoring systems to screen for diabetic peripheral neuropathy. Cochrane Database Syst Rev. 2018;2018(7):CD010974. https://doi.org/10.1002/14651858.CD010974.pub2.
35. Bozkurt AK, Tasci I, Tabak O, Gumus M, Kaplan Y. Peripheral artery disease assessed by ankle-brachial index in patients with established cardiovascular disease or at least one risk factor for atherothrombosis—CAREFUL study: a national, multi-center, cross-sectional observational study. BMC Cardiovasc Disord. 2011;11:4. https://doi.org/10.1186/1471-2261-11-4.
36. National Clinical Guideline Centre (UK). The prevention and management of pressure ulcers in primary and secondary care. London: National Institute for Health and Care Excellence (NICE); 2014. (NICE Clinical Guidelines, No. 179.) 12, Pressure redistributing devices. Available from: https://www.ncbi.nlm.nih.gov/books/NBK333135/.
37. Bashir AZ, Dinkel DM, Pipinos II, Johanning JM, Myers SA. Patient compliance with wearing lower limb assistive devices: a scoping review. J Manip Physiol Ther. 2022;45(2):114–26. https://doi.org/10.1016/j.jmpt.2022.04.003.
38. Chatwin KE, Abbott CA, Boulton AJM, Bowling FL, Reeves ND. The role of foot pressure measurement in the prediction and prevention of diabetic foot ulceration—a comprehensive review. Diabetes Metab Res Rev. 2020;36(4):e3258. https://doi.org/10.1002/dmrr.3258.
39. Reiber GE. Diabetic foot care. Financial implications and practice guidelines. Diabetes Care. 1992;15:29–31.
40. Bakker K, Apelqvist J, Schaper NC. International working group on the diabetic foot editorial board. Practical guidelines on the management and prevention of the diabetic foot 2011. Diabetes Metab Res Rev. 2012;28:225–31.

Chapter 9
Nutritional Management in Diabetic Peripheral Neuropathy

Uma Deaver

Contents

U. Deaver (✉)
Maharishi Markandeshwar Institute of Nursing, MM(DU), Ambala, Haryana, India
e-mail: umadeaver@mmumullana.org

© The Author(s), under exclusive license to Springer Nature Singapore Pte Ltd. 2024

M. Goyal, K. Goyal (eds.), *Rehabilitation in Diabetic Peripheral Neuropathy*,
https://doi.org/10.1007/978-981-97-9290-0_9

9.1 Principle of Nutrition Management

For individuals with diabetic peripheral neuropathy, total calorie intake holds greater importance than the specific proportions of proteins, fats, and carbohydrates in their diet. Any additional calories necessitate extra insulin. A personal scale for weight measurement is as essential for diabetics as checking their urine for sugar.

A diabetic should adhere to a balanced diet that provides sufficient calories to maintain an ideal body weight, which varies based on age, gender, height, and body frame. In obese diabetics, calorie intake should be limited to achieve the ideal body weight; afterward, enough calories should be consumed to maintain a normal weight.

For a same calorie intake, it is advisable to take SIX small meals a day (breakfast-morning snack, lunch, teatime snack, dinner, night snack) rather than three or even one meal [1].

9.2 Goals of Nutrition Management

The goals of nutrition management include encouraging the intake of nutrient-rich foods in suitable portions, achieving personalized glycemic targets, delaying and preventing diabetes complications, and devising dietary plans that consider factors influencing patient preferences. These factors include food preferences, food availability, socioeconomic status, cultural practices, religious beliefs, and geographical location.

9.3 Role of Nutrition Management in DPN

Nutrition plays a crucial role in the management of diabetic peripheral neuropathy (DPN). A well-balanced, a well-planned diet can aid in managing blood sugar levels and decreasing inflammation, and provide essential nutrients that support nerve health. Important points to keep in mind while managing DPN:

- **Blood Sugar Control**: A diet focused on complex carbohydrates, fiber-rich foods, and saturated fats can reduce damage to nerves.
- **Anti-inflammatory Effects**: Foods rich in antioxidants can help reduce inflammation and protect nerves from damage.
- **Nerve Health Nutrients**: Certain nutrients can support nerve function and repair.
- **Weight Management**: A balanced diet can help control weight and reduce the risk of complications associated with obesity, such as nerve compression.
- **Blood Pressure and Cholesterol Control**: A diet low in saturated fats and salt can help control these risk factors.

- **Hydration**: Drinking plenty of water can help to reduce the risk of dehydration-related complications.
- **Avoiding Harmful Substances**: Avoiding excessive alcohol consumption and smoking can prevent further deterioration of nerve function.
- **Individualized Nutrition Plan**: A registered dietitian can provide guidance on portion control, meal timing, and food choices to optimize nerve health.

9.4 Body Weight Management

Research indicates that three-quarters of individuals with diabetes are obese or overweight. Obesity is strongly associated with insulin resistance, characterized by adipose tissue releasing pro-inflammatory adipokines and free fatty acids, which can impede insulin signaling, leading to compensatory hyperinsulinemia and eventually insulin resistance. A weight loss of more than 6 kg with regular physical activity is considered beneficial [2]. An ideal eating pattern is based on different permutations and combination of food items. In India, the four zone eating pattern of Indians is described in (Table 9.1).

Table 9.1 Eating patterns

Eating pattern	Vegetarian foods	Non-vegetarian foods
North Indian	All Dals, Salads made of cucumber, tomatoes, onions, lemon juice, vegetable curries, chickpea curry, raita, whole wheat flatbread (roti), moong dal khichdi, grilled paneertikka	Tandoori chicken (roasted or grilled), Fish curry (salmon or mackeral), chicken soup, chicken tikka, hardboiled egg curry, kebabs (grilled and roasted)lean meat fry, chicken biryani(moderation), chicken salads(add with vegetables)
South Indian	Dosa and idli (made of rice, lentils taken with coconut chutney and sambar), vada, uttapam, Pongal, upma, puliyodere, rasam, vegetable curry.	Grilled or roasted fish, chicken breast, lean cuts of meat, egg whites, dal with meat, grilled chicken or fish salads, soups and steamed chicken or fish.
East Indian	Khichdi, Shak(leafy greens), Dhokla (made of chickpea flour), pithe, tikhur(root vegetable), shukto, chhenepoda, alooposta, a salad made from sprouted beans or lentils, mixed with vegetables.	Spicy pork curry made with Naga chilies and bamboo shoots, light and flavorful fish stew, a traditional drink made from roasted gram flour (sattu), mixed with water, lemon juice, and spices, which is high in protein and fiber.
West Indian	Dhal PuriRoti (flatbread stuffed with seasoned split peas (dhal), Callaloo, Stewed Lentils, Green Banana Curry	Grilled or roasted fish, chicken breast, lean cuts of meat, egg whites, dal with meat, grilled chicken or fish salads, soups and steamed chicken or fish.

9.5 Carbohydrates

The Recommended Dietary Allowance (RDA) mandates a minimum daily intake of 60–65% of total calories must include foods rich in Carbohydrates [3]. This amount is based on the average requirement of glucose needed by the brain. Carbohydrates are of two types: simple and complex (Box 9.1).

Box 9.1 Carbohydrates
Types of carbohydrates

Simple carbohydrates

Simple carbohydrates are rapidly metabolized by the body, making them the fastest source of energy. They consist of sugars such as glucose, fructose, and galactose as well as compounds like sucrose, maltose, and lactose, which are commonly found in fruits, dairy products, and sweeteners.

Complex carbohydrates

Complex carbohydrates include starchy foods that break down into glucose during digestion, such as rice, potatoes, and refined wheat flour. Dietary fiber, a type of non-starchy polysaccharide, refers to carbohydrates that are not digested in the small intestine [3].

9.6 Carbohydrate Counting

Understanding carbohydrate (carb) counting is essential. It involves being conscious of the caloric content of each food item. It's important to know the appropriate caloric intake for every meal, as consuming more than necessary can increase in the blood sugar levels. Person living with diabetes should be proficient in carb counting to implement it at home. This practice serves as a tool for meal planning by monitoring the carbohydrate content in foods, a key nutrient in diet.

The glycemic index (GI) indicates how rapidly a food can increase glucose levels. The foods having carbohydrates possess a GI[4]. Whereas fats and protein do not have a GI, although they can impact blood sugar levels in individuals with diabetes (Box 9.2).

Box 9.2 Glycemic Index Values

Low GI Foods (GI 0–55):

Bulgar, barley, Pasta, parboiled converted) rice, Quinoa, High-fiber bran cereal, Oatmeal, steel-cut or rolled, Carrots, non-starchy vegetables, greens, Apples, oranges, grapefruit, and many other fruits, Most nuts, legumes, and beans, Milk, and yogurt

Moderate GI Foods (GI 56–69):

Pita bread, rye bread, Couscous Brown rice, Raisins

High GI Foods (GI 70 and higher):

White bread and bagels, processed cereals and instant oatmeal, including bran flakes, snack foods, Potatoes, White rice, Honey, Sugar [4]

Low glycemic index (GI) foods cause a gradual increase in blood glucose levels, while high GI foods cause a rapid increase. The GI range from score 0 to 100 with pure glucose having the highest GI value of 100 [4].

9.7 Glycemic Index Values

A glycemic index GI value shows how rapidly particular carbohydrate containing foods turn into sugar. The Physical form (Coarse or fine) or Serving mode (Raw or Cooked) of foods also influence the glycemic index values.

9.8 Protein

The RDA for protein intake can be summarized as follows:

- Protein should contribute to 15–20% of total daily caloric intake.
- Cconsume 1 g of protein per kilogram of present body weight.
- For individuals who are obese, base protein intake on 1 g per kilogram of ideal body weight.
- Ensure that 50% of daily protein intake comes from high-quality, class 1 protein sources.

Class 1 source are foods that contain essential amino acids such as meat, poultry, fish, eggs, milk, cheese, and soya.

Class 2 protein sources are foods that lack one or more essential amino acids, including legumes, pulses, and cereals.

A deficiency in any single amino acid can be remedied by combining foods that complement each other's amino acid profiles. For example, combining idli or dosa with dal, paneer, or yogurt, or pairing rice or roti with dal or paneer can help ensure a balanced intake of essential amino acids.

9.9 Fat

The RDA for fat intake can be summarized as follows:

- 25–35% of total fat intake must be in daily meals.
- Limit saturated fat intake to less than 7% of total daily calories.
- Include up to 10% of daily calories from polyunsaturated fats.
- Incorporate up to 20% of daily calories from monounsaturated fats.

9.10 Total Energy Requirement

Total energy requirement refers to the amount of energy, measured in calories or kilojoules, which an individual needs to maintain their body weight. This requirement is influenced by factors such as age, gender, weight, height, and activity level. Calculating total energy requirement is important for developing personalized nutrition plans and ensuring individuals meet their energy needs for optimal health and performance.

To estimate total energy requirement (kcal/day) using the Harris-Benedict equation is basal metabolic rate (BMR) × physical activity level (PAL). The equations to calculate BMR for men is 88.36 + (13.39 × weight in kg) + (4.79 × height in cm)–(5.68 × age in years) and for women is 447.59 + (9.25 × weight in kg) + (3.09 × height in cm)–(4.33 × age in years).

The criteria for the PAL value is based on the individual's activity level which is given below:

- Sedentary (little or no exercise) = 1.2
- Lightly active (light exercise/sports 1–3 days/week) = 1.375
- Moderately active (moderate exercise/sports 3–5 days/week) = 1.55
- Very active (hard exercise/sports 6–7 days a week) = 1.725
- Super active (very hard exercise and physical job or 2 × training) = 1.9

Finally, to calculate the total energy requirement in kilocalories per day, multiply the BMR by the PAL [5].

For example: A 55-year Mr. X is 60 kgs with height 150 cms and has a physical activity level is little.

BMR = 88.36 + (13.39 × 60) + (4.79 × 150)–(5.68 × 55).

=88.36 + 803.4 + 718.5–312.4 = **1297.86** K Cals/day.

The TER for Mr. X = BMR × PAL.

1297.86 × 1.2 = 1557 K Cals.

9.11 Vitamins and Minerals

Nerves are vital for transmitting signals in the body, and specific nutrients are crucial for their health and function. Essential vitamins and minerals that promote nerve health include

(a) **B Vitamins**:

- **Vitamin B12 (Cobalamin)** is essential for the maintenance of myelin, a protective sheath that surrounds nerves. A deficiency in vitamin B12 can lead to nerve damage and neuropathy. Good sources of vitamin B12 include poultry products, dairy products, and fortified cereals.
- Certain drugs may lead to a B-12 deficiency, such as Tab Metformin [5]
- **B6 (Pyridoxine)**: Vitamin B6 plays a role in producing neurotransmitters, crucial for nerve signaling and is also involved in myelin formation. Dietary sources of vitamin B6 include white meat, seafood, beans, and bananas [6].

(b) **Vitamin D**: Vitamin D is important for nerve health as it plays a role in nerve growth and function. It also has anti-inflammatory effects, which can help protect nerves from damage. Good food sources of vitamin D include fatty fish, eggs, and fortified dairy products. Sunlight exposure is also a natural source of vitamin D [7]

(c) **Vitamin C and E**: Antioxidants, such as vitamins C and E, and beta-carotene, protect nerves from oxidative stress, which can damage nerve cells.

(d) **Omega-3 Fatty Acids**: These are found in fatty fish (salmon, mackerel), flaxseeds, and walnuts and have anti-inflammatory properties that can help protect nerves from damage. Fatty acids consisting of eicosapentaenoic acid (EPA) and docosahexaenoic acid (DHA) provide the brain's required nutrition and reduce blood pressure to adjust glucose rates [8]

- Use 1–2 Tbs. of flaxseed daily
- 3–4 oz. of fatty fish at least 2 times per week.
- 3 oz. of walnuts a day Pittas et al. [8]

(e) **Magnesium**:

Magnesium plays a role in nerve function and can help prevent nerve hyper excitability, which is common in neuropathy. Good sources of magnesium include nuts, seeds, whole grains, and leafy green vegetables [9].

(f) **Alpha-Lipoic Acid**:

Alpha-lipoic acid is a powerful antioxidant that can help protect nerves from damage and improve nerve function. It is found in small amounts in foods like spinach, broccoli, and potatoes but is often taken as a supplement for neuropathy [10].

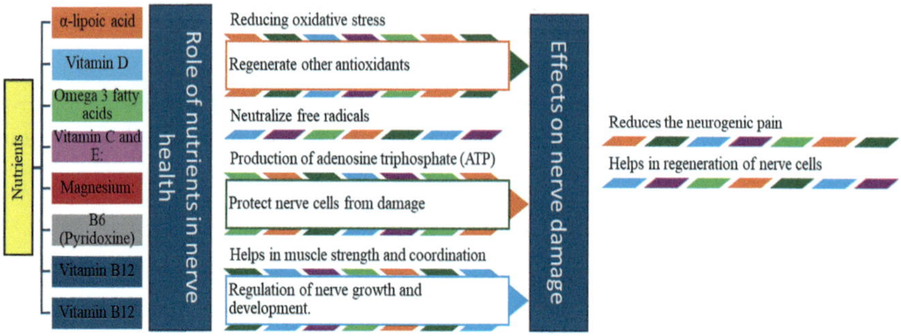

Fig. 9.1 horizontal flow chart showing the role of nutrients in nerve health and its effect on nerve damage

(g) **Acetyl-L-Carnitine:**

Acetyl-L-carnitine is an amino acid that can aid to improve nerve function and lessen the pain in people with neuropathy. It is found in small amounts in red meat and dairy products but is often taken as a supplement for neuropathy. Acetyl-L-carnitine must be avoided people living with diabetes are using warfarin (Coumadin, Jantoven), a blood-thinning medication Additionally, individuals with hypothyroidism or a seizure history should be cautious, as acetyl-L-carnitine may exacerbate these conditions [11].

Figure 9.1 depicts a horizontal flow chart showing the role of nutrients in nerve health and its effect on nerve damage in a nutshell.

9.12 Fibers and Antioxidants

Enhance antioxidant intake by consuming a minimum of five servings of fruits and vegetables daily. Incorporate foods that are slowly metabolized, such as fruits, vegetables, nuts, and legumes, into your diet (Box 9.3).

Box 9.3 Fiber-rich foods

Complex carbohydrates are fibers or molecules made up of long chains of sugar molecules, also known as polysaccharides.

Whole grains: Foods like oats, brown rice, whole wheat, and barley

Fruits: Apples, bananas, oranges, berries, and pears

Vegetables: Broccoli, carrots, spinach, kale, and sweet potatoes are high in fiber.

Legumes: Lentils, chickpeas, black beans, and peas

Nuts and seeds: Almonds, chia seeds, flaxseeds, and sunflower seeds

Whole grain breads and cereals: Look for products that list whole grains as the first ingredient for the most fiber.

Popcorn: Air-popped popcorn is a whole grain and a good source of fiber.

Oatmeal: A bowl of oatmeal is a great way to start your day with a healthy dose of fiber [12].

9.13 Nuts and Seeds

Nuts qualify as sources of the macro mineral elements and unsaturated fats to build the strengthened neuron system and flexible muscles. Such foods also include proteins and carbs that improve brain functions that aid to get rid of neuropathy. Nuts are proven to be taken with vegans and gluten-tolerant people. So, may choose any kind of seeds to provide organisms with healthy proteins and lipids for anti-inflammatory and antibacterial protection abilities. Increase raw nuts and seeds in daily dietary formula to avoid neuropathy progress [13].

9.14 Meal Planning and Management

Meal planning is crucial for ensuring a well-rounded diet, especially for individuals with diabetic peripheral neuropathy (DPN). Meal planning and discussed below:

Control portion sizes: Pictures 9.1 and 9.2 shows the portion sizes, to ensure you're selecting the right amount of each food intake.

Limit added sugars and refined carbs: Foods high in added sugars and refined carbohydrates can cause blood sugar spikes. Limit your intake of sugary drinks, sweets, and processed foods.

Add protein in every meal: Protein can help you feel full and satisfied, and it can help stabilize blood sugar levels. Include lean protein sources such as chicken, fish, tofu, and legumes in your meals.

Don't skip meals: Skipping meals can lead to blood sugar.

Fluctuations: Regular meals and snacks throughout the day help in maintaining a steady blood sugar levels.

Stay hydrated: Drinking plenty of fluids throughout the day help in staying hydrated. Limit sugary drinks and opt for water, herbal tea, or other low-calorie beverages.

Plan ahead: Plan your meals and snacks ahead of time as you make healthier choices and avoid last-minute less healthy options.

Control Portion Sizes

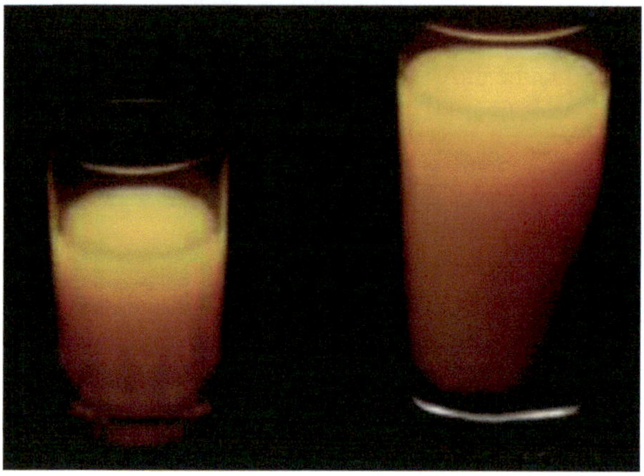

Picture 9.1 Smaller glass is right

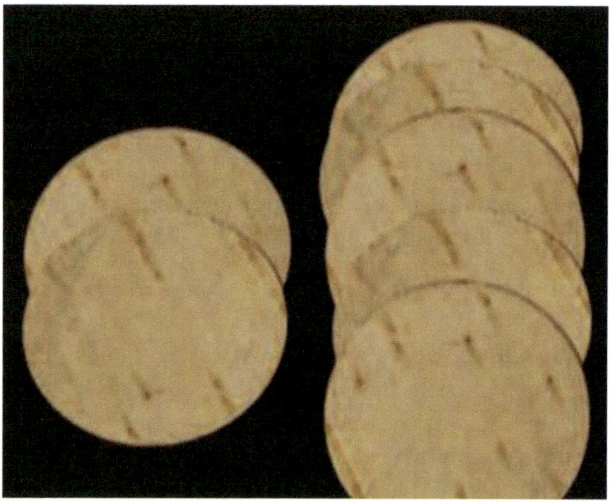

Picture 9.2 Lesser amount is right

9.15 Diet Plan

To make a diabetic diet plan, 60–65% of total calories must include foods rich in carbohydrates, 10–15% of total calories must include foods rich in protein, and 20–25% of total calories must include foods rich in fats.

Example A diabetic diet plan of 1500 kcals /day will be as follows: the total carbohydrate required will be 1500 × 60/100 = 900 Cals. (1 calorie of carbohydrate is equal to 4 g, hence 900 cals/4 g = 225 g of carbohydrate), the total protein required

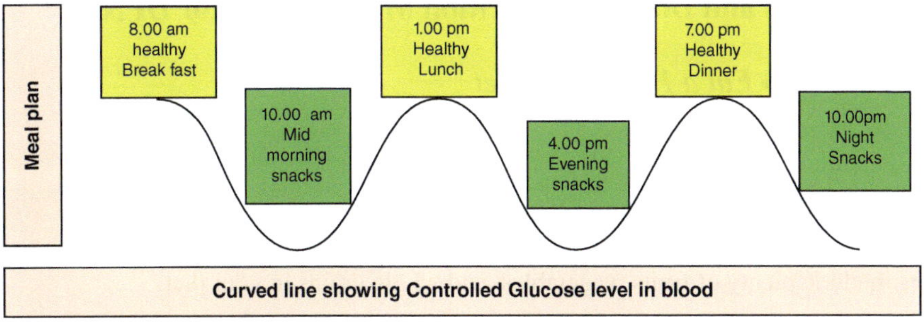

Fig. 9.2 shows the curved line of controlled glucose level in blood

Table 9.2 Diet plan for 1500 K calories

Time	Food items	Quantity	K Calories
6 am	Coffee with milk without sugar	100 ml	65
8 am	Chapati	2	170
	Vegetable curry	½ cup	30
	Egg	1	85
10 am	Green tea	100 ml	
	Boiled groundnut	30 numbers	72
1 pm	Rice	1 cup	170
	Chapati	2	170
	Sambar with vegetables	½ cup pulses	85
	Curd	½ cup	30
	Salads	1 cup	110
4 pm	Fruits	1	40
	Tea with milk without sugar		65
8 pm	Chapati	2	170
	Vegetable curry	½ cup	30
	Mixed vegetable salad	1 cup	48
	Curd	1 cup	30
10 pm	Milk	100 ml	130
		Total	**1500**

will be 1500 × 10/100 = 150 Cals (1 calorie of protein has 4 g), hence 150 cals /4 g = 37.5 g of protein.

Total fat required will be 1500 × 20/100 = 300 cals (1 calorie of protein has 9 g, hence 300 Cals/9 g = 33 g of fat.

Therefore, people living with diabetes with normal BMI must be advised to make a diet plan which should be three meals and three snacks including 225 g of carbohydrate, 37.5 g of protein, and 33 g of fat as shown in Fig. 9.2. Table 9.2 illustrates the diet plan for 1500 K calories [14].

9.16 Do's and Dont's of Nutrition Management for DPN

9.16.1 Do Eat a Healthful Diet

To maintain blood sugar levels as close to normal as possible.

- Eat more frequent, smaller meals.
- Count carbohydrates.
- Include plenty of fruits, vegetables, and whole grains in your diet.

9.16.2 Do Include Food Containing Vitamin B12

To prevent or alleviate peripheral neuropathy caused by vitamin B12 deficiency:

- Consume foods rich in vitamin B12, such as red meat, dairy, fish, eggs, and poultry.
- Consider taking vitamin B12 supplements if needed.

9.16.3 Do Include Foods Containing Lipoic Acid

Lipoic acid deficiency can potentially alleviate diabetic neuropathy, consider the following:

- Ensure adequate intake of lipoic acid, a fatty acid and antioxidant.
- Lipoic acid plays a role in converting blood sugar into energy.
- While most healthy individuals have sufficient lipoic acid, people with diabetes may have low levels.
- Low levels of lipoic acid can contribute to diabetic neuropathy.

9.16.4 Don't Skip Meals

To prevent hypoglycemia in individuals with diabetic neuropathy:

- Enjoy smaller, more frequent meals.
- Avoid skipping meals.
- Check blood sugar levels regularly.

9.16.5 Don't Drink Too Much Alcohol

Follow these guidelines regarding alcohol consumption:

- Limit alcohol intake, as it is toxic to nerves and can worsen neuropathy symptoms.
- Excessive alcohol consumption can lower vitamin B12 levels.
- Alcohol is detrimental to blood sugar control due to its empty calories.
- Be cautious with alcohol on an empty stomach, as it can lead to hypoglycemia, especially if you are taking insulin.

9.16.6 Don't Eat Refined Grains

To improve blood sugar regulation:

- Avoid refined grains found in "white" products like white rice, white bread, and white pasta.
- Opt for whole grains such as brown rice, whole wheat bread, and whole wheat pasta.
- Whole grains contain essential B vitamins and fiber, which are beneficial for your diet.
- Refined grains can make it challenging to regulate blood sugar levels, which can worsen diabetic neuropathy.

9.16.7 Don't Include Gluten Containing Foods

For individuals with gluten sensitivity affecting neuropathy symptoms, consider the following:

- Be cautious with whole grains containing gluten, such as wheat, rye, barley, and oats.
- Gluten sensitivity can exacerbate peripheral neuropathy symptoms.
- Some people may experience neuropathy symptoms when consuming foods containing gluten.

Consider testing for celiac disease if you suspect gluten sensitivity. Many individuals with celiac disease are unaware of their condition [12, 15].

9.17 Future Directions in Nutrition Management of DPN

- Carry a chewable sweet with you, to avoid hypoglycemic attack
- Drink lots of fluids if you suffer with diarrhea to avoid ketoacidosis and coma stage
- Discipline yourself during festivals, celebrations at home or outside
- Know your amount of food to be taken
- Try taking boiled or steamed food instead of fried foods
- Be strict to yourself even if people force
- Try to understand which foods increases your blood sugar level and avoid them as much as possible.

9.18 Home Remedies for Glycemic Control

Foods	Properties
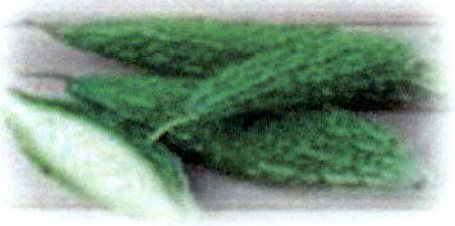	KARELA: Bitter melon's lectin reduces blood sugar and suppresses appetite like insulin, but excessive intake can cause abdominal pain, diarrhea, headache, fever, coma, and worsen low blood sugar [16, 17].
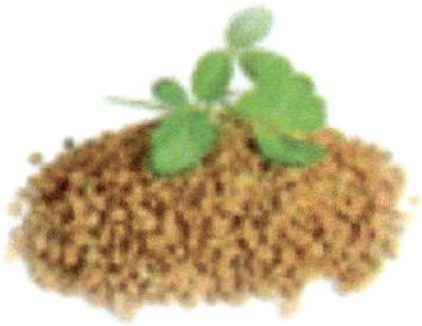	Fenugreek seeds' fiber and compounds slow carb and sugar absorption, reducing post-meal blood sugar spikes when 15 g of powdered seeds are added to a meal for those with type 2 diabetes [18]
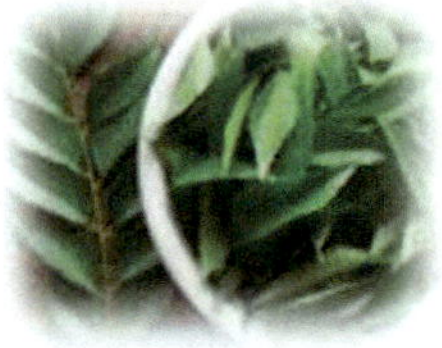	Curry leaves promote weight loss, aid digestion, relieve nausea, fight bacteria, benefit diabetics and eyesight, reduce stress, and heal wounds and skin issues [19].
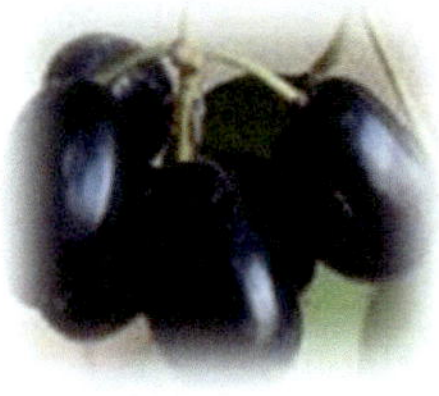	Jamun fruit helps improve blood sugar control, with its pulp and seed both beneficial for diabetes. Consuming 10 g of Jamun seed powder daily can help reduce fasting blood glucose levels [20].

Research Study 1 According to study conducted by AbdelRahman and Hacksaw [21], neuropathic pain affects 7–10% of the population and is often ineffectively and incompletely treated. Patients often turn to "nutraceuticals" in their quest to self-treat neuropathic pain, using readily available supplements. Common choices include vitamins like B and D, trace minerals such as zinc and magnesium, and herbal remedies like curcumin and St. John's Wort [22].

Research Study 2 Hiyoshi et al. [23] examined the effects of postprandial hyperglycemia and postprandial hypertriglyceridemia in individuals with T2DM. The study illustrated how glucose spikes in these patients can lead to vascular injury, causing damage to blood vessels and potentially leading to atherosclerosis. This mechanism is marked by elevated lipid per oxidation, platelet coagulation, and generation of reactive oxygen species (ROS). The research indicated that lowering postprandial glucose levels can aid in decreasing the occurrence of retinopathy and nephropathy in PLD. Furthermore, other factors such as hyperglycemic-induced glomerular hyper filtration, overweight, tobacco use, abnormal lipid levels, extent of protienuria, and dietary aspects might be responsibility in the development of diabetic nephropathy in these patients [16].

9.19 Conclusion

In conclusion, effective nutrition management plays a crucial role in the prevention and management of diabetes peripheral neuropathy. A diet rich in nutrients such as antioxidants, B vitamins, and omega-3 fatty acids can help mitigate oxidative stress, reduce inflammation, and support nerve function. Additionally, maintaining stable blood sugar levels through carbohydrate monitoring and portion control is essential in preventing nerve damage. Patient education and personalized dietary plans are key components in empowering individuals with diabetes to make informed choices and improve their quality of life. Further research and collaboration between healthcare professionals are needed to develop comprehensive strategies for managing diabetes peripheral neuropathy through nutrition.

Self-Assessment

1. Blood sugar control is influenced by the composition, timing, and portion sizes of meals. True/ False
2. A personal weighing scale is as indispensable to a diabetic as is examination of the urine for sugar. True/ False
3. Certain drugs may lead to a B-12 deficiency, including: Tab Metformin True /False
4. Carry a chewable sweet with you, to avoid hypoglycemic attack. True /False

References

1. Leech RM, Worsley A, Timperio A, McNaughton SA. Understanding meal patterns: definitions, methodology and impact on nutrient intake and diet quality. Nutr Res Rev. 2015;28(1):1–21.
2. Cox CE. Role of physical activity for weight loss and weight maintenance. Diabetes Spectr. 2017;30(3):157–60.
3. Carbohydrate recommendations [Internet]. Medicine LibreTexts. Libretexts; 2020 [cited 2024 Mar 20]. Available from: https://med.libretexts.org/Courses/Metropolitan_State_University_of_Denver/Introduction_to_Nutrition_(Diker)/04%3A_Carbohydrates/4.5%3A_Carbohydrate_Recommendations.
4. Carbohydrates and the glycaemic index [Internet]. Gov.au. [cited 2024 Mar 20]. Available from: https://www.betterhealth.vic.gov.au/health/healthyliving/carbohydrates-and-the-glycaemic-index.
5. Glycemic index and diabetes [Internet]. Medlineplus.gov. [cited 2024 Mar 20]. Available from: https://medlineplus.gov/ency/patientinstructions/000941.htm.
6. Thomas N. A practical guide to diabetes mellitus. 8th ed. New Delhi: Jaypee Brothers Medical; 2018.
7. Calderón-Ospina CA, Nava-Mesa MO. B Vitamins in the nervous system: current knowledge of the biochemical modes of action and synergies of thiamine, pyridoxine, and cobalamin. CNS Neurosci Ther. 2020;26(1):5–13.
8. Pittas AG, Dawson-Hughes B, Sheehan P, Ware JH, Knowler WC, Aroda VR, Brodsky I, Ceglia L, Chadha C, Chatterjee R, Desouza C, Dolor R, Foreyt J, Fuss P, Ghazi A, Hsia DS, Johnson KC, Kashyap SR, Kim S, LeBlanc ES, Lewis MR, Liao E, Neff LM, Nelson J, O'Neil P, Park J, Peters A, Phillips LS, Pratley R, Raskin P, Rasouli N, Robbins D, Rosen C, Vickery EM, D2d Research Group. Vitamin D supplementation and prevention of type 2 diabetes. N Engl J Med. 2019;381(6):520–30.
9. Simopoulos AP. Omega-3 fatty acids in inflammation and autoimmune diseases. J Am Coll Nutr. 2002;21(6):495–505.
10. Zhang J, Zhang B, Zhang J, Lin W, Zhang S. Magnesium promotes the regeneration of the peripheral nerve. Front Cell Dev Biol. 2021;9:717854.
11. Viana MDM, Lauria PSS, de Lima AA, Opretzka LCF, Marcelino HR, Villarreal CF. Alpha-lipoic acid as an antioxidant strategy for managing neuropathic pain. Antioxidants (Basel). 2022;11(12):2420.
12. Gonçalves B, Pinto T, Aires A, Morais MC, Bacelar E, Anjos R, et al. Composition of nuts and their potential health benefits—an overview. Food Secur. 2023;12(5):942.
13. Di Stefano G, Di Lionardo A, Galosi E, Truini A, Cruccu G. Acetyl-L-carnitine in painful peripheral neuropathy: a systematic review. J Pain Res. 2019;12:1341–51.
14. Food portions: Choosing just enough for you [Internet]. National Institute of Diabetes and Digestive and Kidney Diseases. NIDDK – National Institute of Diabetes and Digestive and Kidney Diseases; 2024 [cited 2024 Aug 5]. Available from: https://www.niddk.nih.gov/health-information/weight-management/just-enough-food-portions.
15. Berkow SE, Barnard N. Vegetarian diets and weight status. Nutr Rev. 2006;64(4):175–88.
16. Alarim RA, Alasmre FA, Alotaibi HA, Alshehri MA, Hussain SA. Effects of the ketogenic diet on glycemic control in diabetic patients: meta-analysis of clinical trials. Cureus. 2020;12(10):e10796.
17. Joseph B, Jini D. Antidiabetic effects of *Momordica charantia* (bitter melon) and its medicinal potency. Asian Pac J Trop Dis. 2013;3(2):93–102.
18. Ranade M, Mudgalkar N. A simple dietary addition of fenugreek seed leads to the reduction in blood glucose levels: A parallel group, randomized single-blind trial. Ayu [Internet]. 2017;38(1):24. Available from: http://dx.doi.org/10.4103/ayu.ayu_209_15.
19. Kubala J. 9 Impressive curry benefits [Internet]. Healthline 2020 [cited 2024 Aug 5]. Available from: https://www.healthline.com/nutrition/curry-benefits.

20. Kapoor MS. 9 Fruits that protect against diabetes [Internet]. Practocom Practo; 2015 [cited 2024 Mar 20]. Available from: https://www.practo.com/healthfeed/9-fruits-that-protect-against-diabetes-3978/post.
21. Abdelrahman KM, Hackshaw KV. Nutritional supplements for the treatment of neuropathic pain. Biomedicines. 2021;9(6):674.
22. Boers HM, MacAulay K, Murray P, Dobriyal R, Mela DJ, Spreeuwenberg MAM. Efficacy of fibre additions to flatbread flour mixes for reducing post-meal glucose and insulin responses in healthy Indian subjects. Br J Nutr. 2017;117(3):386–94.
23. Hiyoshi T, Fujiwara M, Yao Z. Postprandial hyperglycemia and postprandial hypertriglyceridemia in type 2 diabetes. J Biomed Res. 2017;33(1):1–16.

Chapter 10
Diabetic Foot

Sunita Gupta, Aditi Dabhra, and Sanjeev Gupta

Contents

S. Gupta
Department of Internal Medicine, Maharishi Markandeshwar Institute of Medical Sciences and Research, MMDU, Ambala, India

A. Dabhra · S. Gupta (✉)
Department of Dermatology, Maharishi Markandeshwar Institute of Medical Sciences and Research, MMDU, Ambala, India

© The Author(s), under exclusive license to Springer Nature Singapore Pte Ltd. 2024

M. Goyal, K. Goyal (eds.), *Rehabilitation in Diabetic Peripheral Neuropathy*,
https://doi.org/10.1007/978-981-97-9290-0_10

10.1 Introduction

Diabetes mellitus (DM) is a progressive metabolic disorder marked by a state of hyperglycemia, mostly due to insulin resistance or insulin deficiency. Hyperglycemia that has been present for a long period of time is the cause of a significant number of complications. The term "diabetic foot" refers to a variety of complications pertaining to the foot that may develop in people who have diabetes. Feet are more prone to trauma due to several factors related to their complex structure, weight-bearing function, exposed location, and limited protection. Diabetic neuropathy which is one among the serious complications of diabetes can have a direct and significant impact on the development of diabetic foot as injuries may go unnoticed.

The diabetic foot ulcer is most fatal, most dreadful, least diagnosed, most frequently mistreated, and least effectively managed diabetic complication. Charcot neuroarthropathy, foot ulcerations, infections, and necrosis all contribute to the severe and potentially life-threatening consequences of lower limb amputation. While it is not possible to prevent the majority of these complications, their occurrence can be mitigated through appropriate management. Diabetes is a prevalent primary factor leading to non-traumatic amputations of the lower extremities (L.E.A.s). The impact of lower extremity amputation on an individual patient is very enormous. Hence, amputation is the last resort of an unsalvageable limb.

Accurately assessing the likelihood of amputation in individuals diagnosed with diabetic foot ulcers is critical to prevent the severe morbidity and mortality associated with the condition and to ensure that the limb can be preserved through appropriate management. It is, therefore, very important to prevent diabetic foot, given the detrimental effects it has on patients' quality of life and the financial strain it places on the healthcare system.

10.2 Definition

Diabetic foot is defined as the presence of ulceration, infection, and/or destruction of deep tissues associated with neurologic abnormalities and various degrees of peripheral arterial disease (PAD) in the lower limb in individuals with diabetes [1].

American Diabetes Association defines chronic diabetic foot ulcer as a wound failing to heal after 4 weeks.

10.3 Epidemiology

Diabetes mellitus is projected by the World Health Organization to rank as the seventh most prevalent cause of mortality on a global scale by the year 2030 [2].

In the overall population of diabetics, foot ulceration occurs at a rate of 4–10%; however, it is lower (1.5–3.5%) in younger patients and greater (5–10%) in older ones. People with type 1 diabetes or type 2 diabetes have a foot ulceration incidence rate of less than 1%–3.6% per year. Although the current lifetime risk for this consequence ranges from 19% to 34%, only approximately 5% of diabetic people have a history of ulceration of foot.

Foot problems are mostly common in some ethnic groups than others. Compared to White Americans, those of African American, Native American, and Hispanic descent have a greater chance of developing foot ulcers [3].

Following the initial assessment, it is observed that within a time frame of 6–18 months, a considerable proportion (10–15%) of foot ulcers resolve, while a mere 5–24% necessitate amputation. In specialized tertiary centers, outcome data indicates that around 77% of diabetic foot ulcers resolve within 1 year [4].

Amputation represents the primary detrimental consequence of foot ulceration. The rates of non-traumatic lower extremity amputations in those with diabetes remain 10–20 times greater compared to those without diabetes. Patients diagnosed with diabetes account for an estimated 40–70% of all non-traumatic lower limb amputations. Ischemia and infection are the leading causes of amputation in patients with diabetes. Critical limb ischemia or nonhealing foot ulcers account for amputation in 30–50% of patients with diabetes, while infection is responsible for amputation in 50–70% [5].

10.4 Economic Aspects

Most studies on foot ulcers focus on direct expenditures such as hospital bills, antibiotic medications, diagnostic and therapeutic interventions, bandages, and offloading devices. In addition to direct costs, there is are also indirect costs, such as lost income, early retirement, and rehabilitation expenditures, are harder to assess. Quality of life is a crucial factor for foot ulcer patients that cannot be quantified economically. Foot ulcers can impede the performance of daily tasks and leisure activities for individuals. Patients with foot ulceration or amputation experience higher rates of depression and lower quality of life compared to those without any foot problems.

A 1994–2000 study found that diabetic foot ulcers without lower limb amputations costs US$993–US$17,519. European studies estimated that diabetic foot ulcer patients spent US$13,561 yearly on direct and indirect care. A 2017 study found that diabetic foot ulcer treatment costs US$1960 in India [6].

10.5 Etiology and Risk Factors for Foot Ulceration

There are two primary factors that lead to the formation of diabetic foot ulcers in individuals with diabetes (Flowchart 10.1) (Table 10.1).

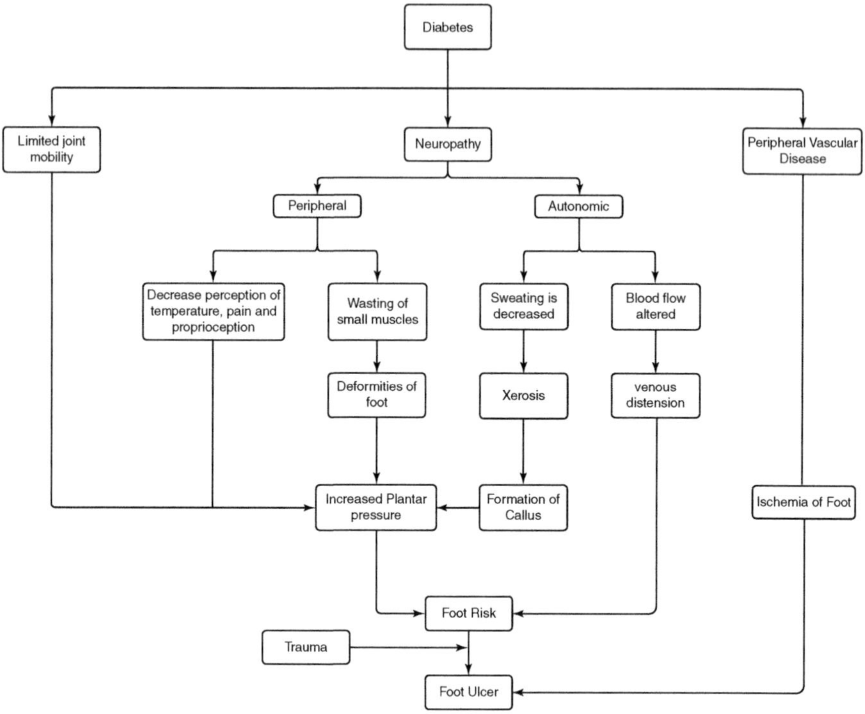

Flowchart 10.1 Depicting foot ulceration pathway

Table 10.1 Showing risk factors for foot ulceration

General/systemic causes	Local causes
Uncontrolled hyperglycemia	Structural foot deformity
Blindness or visual loss	Callus
Chronic kidney disease	Trauma
Duration of diabetes	Peripheral neuropathy
Peripheral vascular disease	Limited joint mobility
Older age	Prolonged pressure
	History or prior ulcer/amputation

1. Causative factors

   A. *Peripheral neuropathy*—It is the primary and most critical cause.

      (a) Sensory neuropathy typically progresses to a depth of at least 50% prior to the onset of protective sensation loss. This leads to loss of protective function, loss of pain, pressure, and proprioception increasing the risk of foot ulcers due to physical and thermal damage.

      (b) Motor neuropathy affects leg muscles, causing aberrant bone protrusion, altered foot architecture, and deformities including hammer toe and hallux rigidus.

(c) Autonomic neuropathy, also known as auto sympathectomy causes xerosis, decreased sweat, and increased secondary capillary refill due to arteriovenous fissures making the foot vulnerable to minor trauma [7].

B. *High foot plantar pressure*—It is the second-most important factor for diabetic foot ulcer. The issue stems from joint mobility limits (subtalar, ankle, and first metatarsophalangeal joints) and foot abnormalities. Within 2.5 years, 28% of peripheral neuropathy patients with elevated plantar pressure will develop foot ulcers compared to those without [7].
C. *Trauma*—Recurring trauma, footwear friction (21%), foot injuries (11%), tinea pedis leading to cellulitis (4%), and nail cut errors (4%) [7].
D. *Diabetic Foot Infections*—DFIs can be induced by various microorganisms, although Staphylococcus aureus is the most commonly found among Gram-positive organisms. Methicillin-resistant Staphylococcus aureus (MRSA) is detected in 16.78%–30% of DFI cases. Eight Most common gram-negative organisms found are Proteus species, *Escheria coli*, Klebsiella, Pseudomonas and Citrobacter species.

2. Contributory factors

(a) *Atherosclerosis*—Atherosclerosis from peripheral vascular disease, particularly in femoropopliteal and tiny blood arteries below the knee, is the primary contributor [7].
(b) *Diabetes*—Diabetes causes intrinsic wound healing challenges, such as collagen cross-linking problems, matrix metalloproteinases dysfunction, and immunologic diseases, particularly decreased polymorphonuclear leukocyte activity. Diabetics have an increased risk of onychomycosis and tinea infections, leading to easy skin peeling and infections. In DM, poor acute inflammatory responses and impaired angiogenesis lead to wound healing issues [7].

10.5.1 Risk Factors for Foot Ulceration

1. *Extrinsic Factors*—Walking without footware, inappropriate footwear, accidents and falls, objects inside shoes, sharp injuries or thermal injury.
2. *Intrinsic Factors*—Bony Prominences, Limited mobility of joint, Deformity of Joint, Callus, Fissures, History of past foot surgeries, or Neuro-osteoarthropathic joint.

10.6 Pathophysiology of Diabetic Foot

Diabetic ulcers are caused by metabolic abnormalities, neuropathy, angiopathy, and immune system alterations (Fig. 10.1) (Flowchart 10.2).

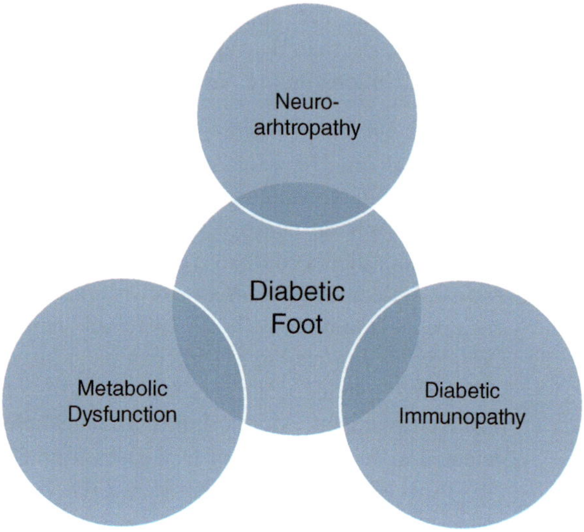

Fig. 10.1 Showing pathophysiological factors leading to diabetic foot

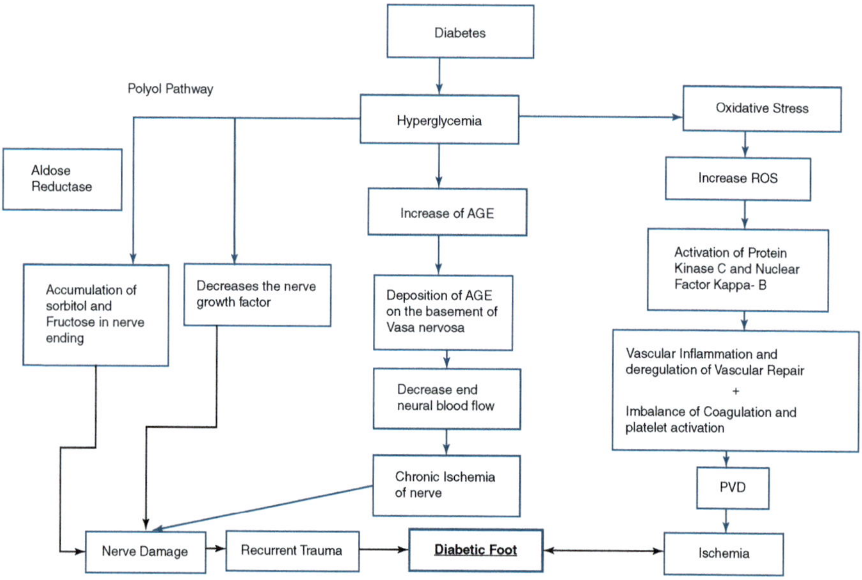

Flowchart 10.2 Showing mechanism of metabolic dysfunction. (*AGE* Advanced Glycation End Products, *ROS* Reactive Oxygen Species, *PVD* Peripheral Vascular Disease)

1. *Metabolic Dysfunction*—Mechanism of metabolic dysfunction, neuropathy, and angiopathy contributing to the foot ulcers is described below (Flowchart 10.2)
2. *Diabetic Immunopathy*—Mechanism of diabetic immunopathy is described in the flow chart below (Flowchart 10.3)
3. *Neuroarthropathy*

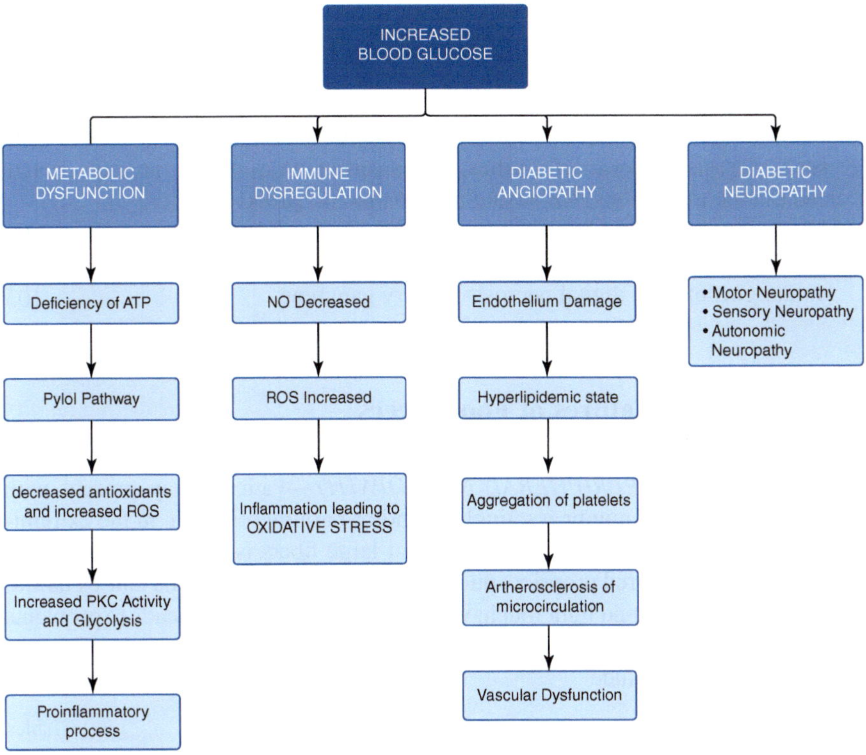

Flowchart 10.3 Showing Pathophysiology of Foot Ulceration. (*ATP* Adenosine Triphosphate, *NO* Nitric Oxide, *ROS* Reactive oxygen species, *PKC* Protein kinase C)

- Charcot neuroarthropathy, also referred to as Charcot foot, is a long-lasting, progressive degenerative condition of the joints that occurs due to impaired sensory innervation of the affected joint.
- Charcot foot is characterized by the presence of soft-tissue edema, bone osteolysis, dislocation and subluxation of joints.
- Under modulated stimulation, proinflammatory proteins manifest unique expression patterns in patients afflicted with Charcot foot. Osteolysis is initiated uncontrollably when proinflammatory cytokines, including interleukin (IL)-1β and tumor necrosis factor-α, are produced.
- The expression of the anti-inflammatory peptides IL-4 and IL-10 is reduced, whereas the expression of receptor activator of nuclear factor (NF)-κB ligand (RANKL) is increased. RAKL facilitates osteoclast maturation via NF-κB activation.
- Charcot foot is characterized by midfoot collapse or "rocker-bottom" foot deformity. Hallux valgus may occur. These abnormalities heighten the vulnerability to repeated ulcerations [8].

10.7 Classification of Foot Ulcers

Diabetic foot is classified into two types:

1. *Neuropathic Foot*—In this neuropathy predominates. Neuropathy leads to fissures, xerosis, various deformities, callus formation at plantar pressure points and plantar ulcerations, bullae and neuropathic (Charcot) joint.
2. *Neuroischemic Foot*—In this type of occlusive vascular disease predominates although neuropathy is present. Ischemia further leads to pain at rest, ulceration on margins of foot, digital necrosis and dry gangrene.

10.8 Clinical Features of Foot Ulcers

1. *SYMPTOMS OF PERIPHERAL NEUROPATHY*—Patients may present with varying degrees of numbness, tingling, and/or burning sensation in the extremities which may be worst at night. Loss of large fibers is reflected in problems with vibration, altered proprioception (which impacts balance and causes numbness and tingling), and light touch, whereas loss of small fibers leads to problems with pain and temperature sensation. Common symptoms of peripheral neuropathy in diabetics include

   (i) Hyperesthesia
   (ii) Hypoesthesia
   (iii) Dysesthesia
   (iv) Paresthesia
   (v) Anhidrosis
   (vi) Radicular pain

2. *SYMPTOMS OF PERIPHERAL ARTERIAL INSUFICIENCY*—The majority of individuals with lower extremity atherosclerotic disease are asymptomatic, although a subset may manifest ischemic symptoms. Symptomatic patients may exhibit

   (i) *Intermittent claudication*—It is indicated by cramping or fatigue of main muscle groups in one or both lower extremities that are reproducible after walking a certain distance. This symptom gains intensity during physical activity until it becomes impracticable to walk; it is alleviated by a brief period of rest. Walking at a faster pace, ascending stairs, or walking incline may hasten the onset of claudication.
   (ii) *Frank ischemia of the foot*—Diabetic individuals frequently experience discomfort, cramping, or weakness in the calves or feet due to a high incidence of tibioperoneal atherosclerotic occlusions.

(iii) *Nonhealing ulceration of the foot*—typically manifests as a region of erythema on the affected area, which subsequently breaks down, leaving an open wound in the skin that is resistant to healing.
(iv) *Ischemic pain at rest*—Pain at rest is less prevalent among individuals with diabetes. A fissure, ulcer, or other breach in the integrity of the skin envelope may serve as the initial indication of perfusion loss.

10.9 Assessment of Diabetic Foot Ulcer

A comprehensive physical examination and medical history should be obtained. Since it is evident that these patients are frequently under evaluated, even when hospitalized, a methodical approach to their comprehensive assessment is necessary. In the medical history, the indications and symptoms of diabetic foot ulcer or any pre-ulcerative lesion should be emphasized. Additionally, symptoms that may suggest peripheral neuropathy or peripheral arterial insufficiency must be investigated (Fig. 10.2).

10.9.1 Past Medical History

The medical history should evaluate the cardiovascular, neurological, renal, and dermatological condition of the patient with diabetes. The patient's present medication regimen and history of antibiotic use should be carefully considered because they may compromise therapy efficacy or cause treatment to be ineffective. Pain should be considered as an unreliable symptom in patients having peripheral neuropathy. The patient should be questioned regarding previous surgical procedures, history of ulcerations, infections, or trauma that occurred at the current site or any other site of infection in the past.

10.9.2 Present History

Constitutional symptoms, including but not limited to fever, nausea, malaise, fatigue, vomiting or shivers, are critical clinical indicators to include in the present medical history when a diabetic foot is infected. The possibility of sepsis or a severe infection exists and must be evaluated. Systemic indications, such as fever and leukocytosis, are not observed in around 50% of diabetic patients who present with a significant infection [9]. Persistent hyperglycemia often serves as the sole indicator of an infection [10]. History of fever, pain, local swelling should be taken.

The history of the wound or infection should include the onset, duration, and appearance before inspection of the area. The depth or size of the ulcer, volume of

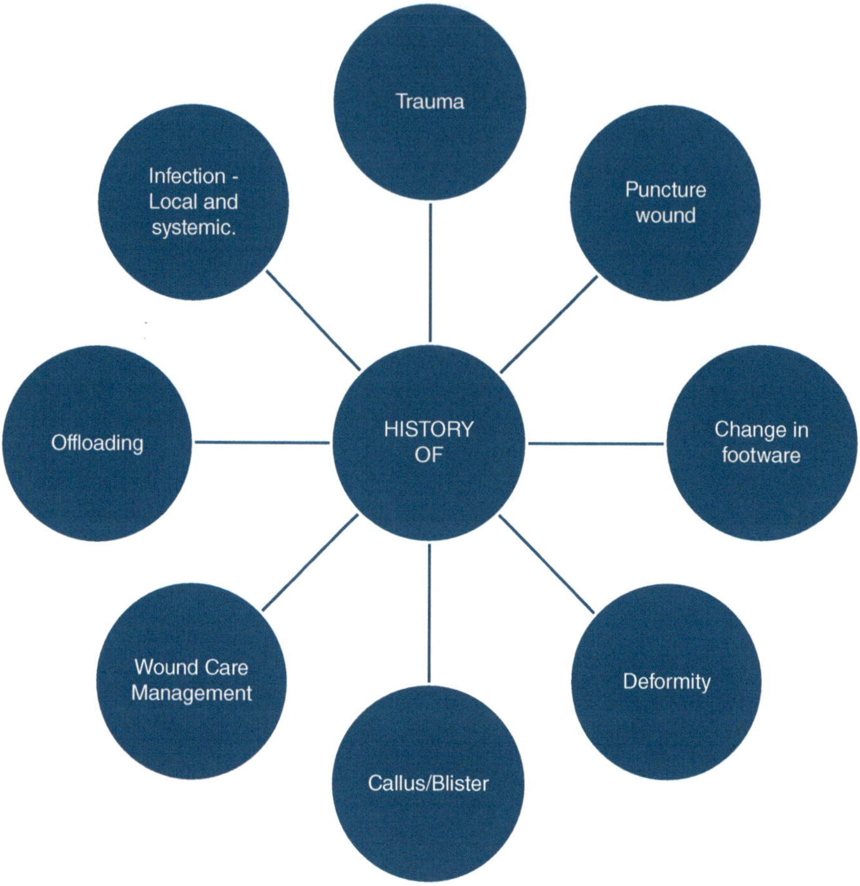
Trauma
Infection -
Local and
systemic.
Puncture
wound
Offloading
HISTORY
OF
Change in
footware
Wound Care
Management
Deformity
Callus/Blister

Fig. 10.2 Depicting points for diagnosis of diabetic foot ulcers or pre-ulcerative lesions

discharge, swelling, color, odor, and extent of infection should be evaluated. To find out if the infection or ulcer has spread to the tendon sheaths, sinuses, bones, or joints, it is necessary to probe the area. The latter are typical routes for proximal and distal infection transmission. It is presumed that the patient has osteomyelitis if bone is exposed until proven differently.

10.10 Clinical Examination of Diabetic Foot

A complete foot examination and pedal inspection are part of the standard clinical examination protocol for all diabetic patients seeing any healthcare provider and should be done annually (Fig. 10.3).

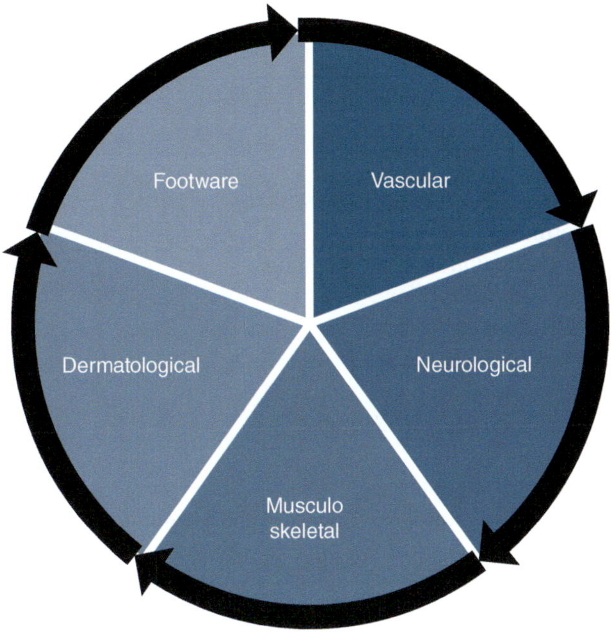

Fig. 10.3 Various examinations for diabetic foot

1. **Vascular examination**—For evaluating blood flow to the lower extremities, a vascular examination is vital in diabetic foot care. Diabetes can lead to peripheral vascular disease, which can impair blood circulation to the feet and increase the risk of ulcers and infections. The assessment includes

   - Peripheral pulse examination—Femoral, popliteal, posterior tibial, and dorsalis pedis
   - Filling time of subpapillary venous plexus—normal <3 s.
   - Venous filling time—normal <20 s.
   - Symptoms of ischemia include cyanosis, redness, swelling.
   - Localized rise in temperature.
   - Changes in the skin—Nail and skin atrophy, wrinkling, sparse pedal hair.

2. **Neurological examination**—Neurologic Examination should include:

   - Vibration perception (using the Tuning fork 128 Hz).
   - Semmes-Weinstein 10-g monofilament for examination of light touch (pressure perception).
   - Cotton wool for light touch.
   - Pinprick for superficial pain.
   - Examination of Vibration Pressure Threshold by Biothesiometer.
   - Examination of temperature sensation.
   - Deep tendon reflexes.

- Ankle (Achilles tendon) reflex.
- Knee (patellar) reflex.
- Babinski test.
- Rhomberg's test.

3. **Musculoskeletal examination**

- Biomechanical abnormalities assessment.
- Bone deformities.
- Hammertoes, bunion or tailor's bunion.
- Flat feet or high-arched feet.
- Charcot deformities.
- Amputations.
- Limited joint mobility.
- Tendo-achilles contractures/equinus.
- Gait evaluation.
- Muscle group strength testing.
- Passive and active, non-weight bearing and weight bearing.
- Foot drop.
- Intrinsic muscle atrophy.
- Assessment of Plantar pressure.
- Treadmill Test.

4. **Dermatological examination**

- Skin appearance—Color, texture, xerosis. A smooth shiny wrinkled skin is characteristic of early changes found in Diabetic foot.
- Signs of Ischemia—Look for blueish discoloration of skin.
- Shin spots.
- Nail deformities—Ingrown nails, onychodystrophy, onychogryphosis.
- Diabetic dermopathy.
- Necrobiosis lipoidica diabeticorum.
- Bullous diabeticorum.
- Granuloma annulare.
- Infection—Note location, size, and depth.
- Web Space Examination—maceration, fissuring, ulceration, interdigital lesions.
- Examination for Tinea pedis and Onychomycosis.
- Look for signs of gangrene.

5. **Footwear examination**

- Shoe type.
- Fit of shoe.
- Patterns of wear.
- Foreign bodies.
- Insoles.
- Orthoses.

Table 10.2 The Meggitt-Wagner classification

Grade	Description of ulcer
Grade 0	Pre ulcerative or post-ulcerative lesion which is completely epithelialized.
Grade 1	Superficial, full in thickness ulcers which is limited to the dermis, not extending up to the subcutis.
Grade 2	Ulcer extending through the subcutis With exposed tendon or bone but without any Osteomyelitis or abscess formation.
Grade 3	Ulcer is deep with osteomyelitis or abscess formation
Grade 4	Localized gangrene of toes or the forefoot.
Grade 5	Extensive gangrene of the foot.

Table 10.3 The University of Texas classification for diabetic foot wounds

	Grade 0	Grade 1	Grade 2	Grade 3
Stage A	Pre-ulcerative or post-ulcerative lesion which is completely epithelialized	Wound is superficial and not involving any tendon, capsule or bone.	Penetrating wound to the tendon or capsule	Penetrating wound to bone or joint
Stage B	Infection present	Infection present	Infection present	Infection present
Stage C	Ischemia present	Ischemia present	Ischemia present	Ischemia present
Stage D	Infection present and ischemia present	Infection present and ischemia present	Infection present and ischemia present	Infection present and ischemia present

10.11 Assessment of Diabetic Foot Ulcer

Various Classifications have been proposed for classification of foot ulcers

- Meggitt-Wagner classification
- University of Texas classification system for diabetic foot wounds

1. *The Meggitt-Wagner classification* [11]—It is the primary and validated categorization for foot ulcers (Table 10.2).
2. *The University of Texas classification system for diabetic foot wounds* [12]—is validated and proposed by the University of Texas. This approach assesses ulcer depth, infection similar to the Meggitt-Wagner classification and ischemia (Table 10.3).

10.12 Investigations for Diabetic Foot

Clinical evaluation, laboratory analyses, imaging studies, and other modalities are commonly employed in diabetic foot investigations to determine the degree of neuropathy, vascular impairment, and tissue damage (Fig. 10.4).

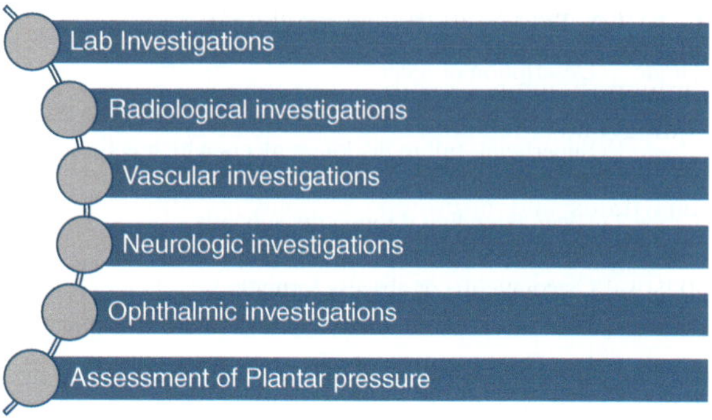

Fig. 10.4 Investigations for diabetic foot

1. **Lab investigations**—In the process of assessing the condition and potential complications of a diabetic foot in a patient, a number of laboratory investigations may prove beneficial. These investigations include:

   - Blood Glucose Levels—fasting and postprandial glucose levels.
   - Hemoglobin A1c (HbA1c)
   - Complete Blood Count (CBC)
   - LFT
   - RFT
   - C-reactive Protein (CRP)
   - Erythrocyte Sedimentation Rate (ESR)
   - Serum Creatinine and Estimated Glomerular Filtration Rate (eGFR)
   - Lipid Profile.
   - Urine Analysis—done for proteinuria, microalbuminuria, and urinary tract infections.
   - Wound Swab Cultures.

2. **Radiological Investigations**—Radiological studies are extremely important for the evaluation and management of diabetic foot problems. When it comes to determining the level of soft tissue and bone involvement, determining the underlying pathology, and directing treatment options, radiological investigations play a particularly important role. In the case of diabetic foot, some typical radiographic investigations include the following:

   - X-rays (Radiography)
   - Computed tomography (CT) Scan)
   - Magnetic resonance imaging (MRI)
   - Bone scintigraphy (Bone Scan)

3. **Vascular investigations**—As decreased blood flow is a substantial risk factor for poor wound healing, tissue necrosis, and amputation, vascular investigations are the most important part of evaluating the vascular state of patients who have issues related to diabetic foot. In order to evaluate the vascular supply of the lower extremities in diabetic foot patients, there are a few different vascular studies that can be utilized:

- Doppler Ultrasound—Ankle-Brachial Index (ABI) and Toe-Brachial Index (TBI)
- Duplex ultrasound
- Magnetic Resonance Angiography (MRA)
- Computed Tomography Angiography (CTA)
- Angiography

4. **Neurological investigations**—Neurological evaluations are critical for determining the functionality of the sensory, motor, and autonomic nervous systems in patients who have complications of diabetic foot. Neuropathy, a prevalent complication of diabetes and a substantial risk factor for foot ulceration and lower extremity amputations, is identified through these tests. A variety of neurological examinations may be utilized to assess diabetic foot neuropathy:
   - Nerve Conduction Studies (NCS)
   - Electromyography (EMG)
   - Quantitative Sensory Testing (QST)
   - Autonomic Function Tests
5. **Ophthalmic Investigations**—They may reflect long standing uncontrolled blood sugar levels in a patient presenting with diabetic foot and therefore help in evaluating chronicity of diabetes. Various investigations for this include
   - Fundus Examination
   - Intraocular Pressure Measurement
   - Fluorescein Angiography
   - Optical Coherence Tomography (OCT)
6. **Assessment of Plantar Foot Pressure**—Plantar pressures are typically measured for footwear insoles and not to diagnose neuropathy, as even patients without neuropathy may have aberrant pressures due to structural deformities. Devices that measure foot pressures during walking or standing can help identify high-pressure points. Various techniques involved include
   - Carbon paper imprint of the feet
   - Podoscope
   - Foam Mark
   - Treadmills
   - Scanners
   - Pressure Insoles.

10.12.1 Diabetic Foot Risk Assessment

Diabetic foot risk assessment (DIAFORA) classification [13] is a recently introduced tool. In comparison to the current classification systems, this one demonstrated comparable or superior accuracy in predicting the lower extremity amputation

Table 10.4 DIAFORA classification for risk assessment of amputation in diabetic foot ulcer patient

Variables	Score
Peripheral neuropathy (Inability to feel monofilament)	+4
Foot deformity (Foot alteration and increasing pressure in > = 1 sites of foot)	+1
Peripheral arterial disease (None or only one foot pulse is Palpable)	+7
Previous DFU/LEA	+3
Multiple DFU (>1 DFU)	+4
Infections (discharge mainly purulent type and any of the local signs of infection)	+4
DFU affects the bone.	+7
Gangrene present. (Wet/Dry)	+10

DFU Diabetic foot ulcer, *LEA* Lower extremity amputations

in patients having diabetic foot ulcers. According to the study, this classification is highly accurate for the lower extremity amputation prediction in patients with diabetic foot ulcer. The eight different variables with their individual score are (Table 10.4).

The subjects can be categorized into three groups:

- <15 points = Risk is low.
- 15–25 points = Risk is medium.
- >25 points = Risk is high.

10.13 Management of Diabetic Foot

Managing diabetic foot requires a multifaceted approach. Here are four pillars for diabetic foot management (Fig. 10.5) (Flowchart 10.4).

10.13.1 Mechanical Control

Mechanical control in diabetic foot management primarily focuses on offloading pressure from areas of the foot that are at risk of developing ulcers or wounds. Mechanical control aims to reallocate pressure away from vulnerable areas to prevent the formation of ulcers and promote healing in existing wounds. Here are some strategies for mechanical control:

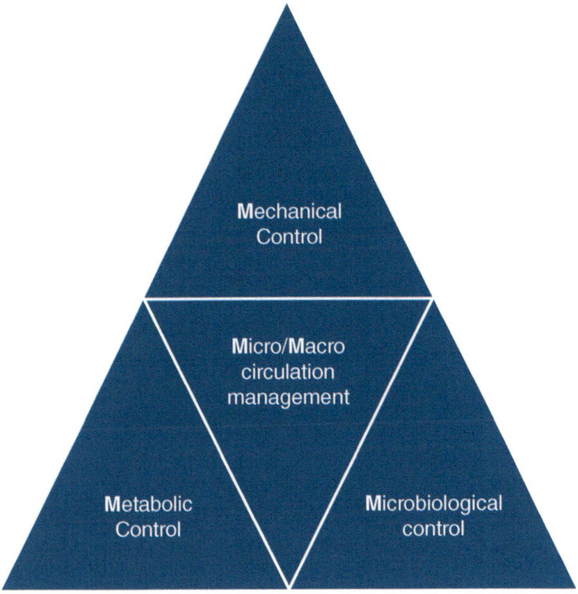

Fig. 10.5 Showing pillars for diabetic foot management

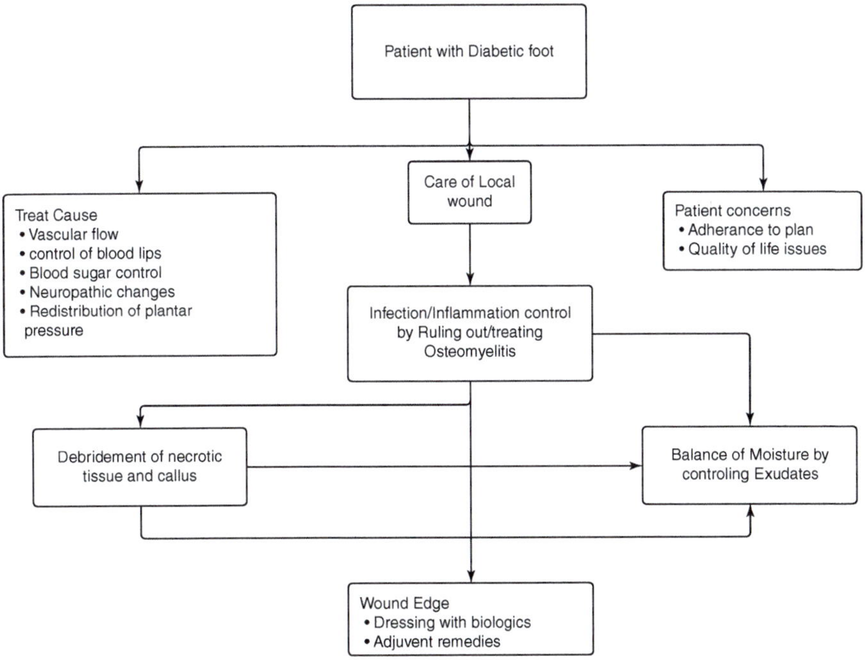

Flowchart 10.4 Showing pathway to assessment/treatment of a patient with diabetic foot ulcer

- *Footwear Modification*—Shoes should fit well, provide adequate support, and have cushioning to reduce pressure on the feet. In some cases, custom-made shoes or orthotic inserts may be necessary to accommodate foot deformities and redistribute pressure evenly.
- *Total Contact Casting (TCC)*—TCC involves the application of a specialized cast that conforms closely to the shape of foot, providing uniform pressure distribution and offloading areas of high pressure. TCC is particularly effective for offloading diabetic foot ulcers and promoting healing.
- *Removable Cast Walkers*—Removable cast walkers, such as controlled ankle motion (CAM) boots, are devices that provide support and offload pressure from the foot while allowing patients to walk. These devices are often used in conjunction with TCC or for individuals who require mobility during the healing process.
- *Pressure-Relieving Insoles and Pads*—Specialized insoles and pads can be placed inside shoes to decrease pressure on specific areas of foot. These may include metatarsal pads, heel cups or cushioned insoles designed to redistribute pressure and provide additional support.
- *Offloading Devices*—Various offloading devices, such as diabetic foot braces or orthotic devices can be used to alleviate pressure from specific areas of the foot. These devices are custom designed to address individual foot deformities and provide support where needed.
- *Regular Foot Monitoring*—Diabetic individuals should perform daily foot inspections to check for any signs of redness, swelling, blisters or other abnormalities. Early detection of problems allows for prompt intervention and prevention of complications.

10.13.2 Micro/Macro Circulation Management

Vascular management in diabetic foot care is essential because diabetes can lead to peripheral arterial disease (PAD). Poor blood circulation can contribute to delay in wound healing, increased risk for infection and higher rates of limb amputation in diabetic individuals. Here are some key aspects of vascular management in diabetic foot care:

- Vascular Assessment—Regular vascular assessments are crucial for diabetic individuals, especially those with known risk factors. Non-invasive tests like ankle-brachial index (ABI), Doppler ultrasound, and toe-brachial index (TBI) are used to evaluate blood flow to the feet and detect any arterial blockages or abnormalities.
- Cardiovascular risk factor reduction—This may involve lifestyle modifications, medications, and interventions to control the blood pressure, cholesterol levels, and blood sugar.
- Revascularization Procedures—Revascularization may be needed to restore blood flow to a limb with severe peripheral arterial disease and critical limb isch-

emia (CLI). Angioplasty, stenting, atherectomy, and bypass surgery can enhance circulation.

10.13.3 Microbiological Control

A prognostic indicator for inadequate wound healing and amputation is the presence of an infection in the lesion [14]. Infections of the diabetic foot are frequently caused by a variety of bacteria, fungi, and occasionally anaerobic organisms as well. Key strategies for microbiological control in diabetic foot care include the following:

- *Antibiotic Therapy*—Specific guidelines regarding the management of the diabetic foot infections have been established by the Infectious Diseases Society of America (IDSA) [15]. The IDSA advises that lesions exhibiting a minimum of two signs or symptoms of inflammation (such as erythema, tenderness, induration or pain) or purulent discharge necessitate treatment. Prior to administering antibiotic treatment, it is recommended to acquire a deep tissue culture by performing curettage or biopsy after debridement.
- Specifically, it is important to refrain from using swab specimens in lesions that have not been sufficiently cleaned and removed of debris. When treating infections which are mild to moderate, aerobic Gram-positive cocci should be focus of the antibiotic treatment. If culture results are not available, it is recommended to use broad-spectrum empiric antibiotics to treat severe infections.
- The IDSA advises a course of antibiotics lasting 1–2 weeks for mild infections and 2–3 weeks for moderate infections to severe infections; however, antibiotic treatment can typically be discontinued once the clinical manifestations of the infection have subsided [13]. In order to avoid the development of antibacterial resistance and other negative treatment outcomes, it is advised to treat clinical diabetic foot infections with narrow-spectrum antibiotics for the shortest possible duration [13].
- *Dressings and topical agents*—The type of wound, lesion characteristics, presence of infection, patient preference, and cost-effectiveness are all important factors that must be taken into account when making a choice for diabetic foot ulcers dressings (Table 10.5).

10.13.4 Metabolic Control

Metabolic control in diabetes pertains to regulation of the blood glucose levels as well as additional metabolic parameters including blood pressure, cholesterol, and weight, with the objectives of averting complications and upholding general well-being. Key components of metabolic control in diabetes include the following:

Table 10.5 Various dressings used in the treatment of diabetic foot ulcer

Type	Actions
Alginates/Carboxymethyl cellulose	Absorption of fluid. Promotion of autolytic debridement. Control of moisture. Conformability to the wound bed. Suitable for heavy exudative wounds
Foams	Highly absorbent Moisture control Suitable for moderately exuding wounds
Honey	Rehydration of wound bed. Promotion of autolytic debridement. Antimicrobial action Used as honey jaggery dressing.
Hydrocolloids	Form a gel when in contact with wound exudate. Facilitates granulation tissue formation. Suitable for low to moderately exuding wounds Can provide some level of protection against bacterial contamination. Promote autolytic debridement
Hydrogels	Cooling and soothing properties Suitable for dry or minimally exuding wounds Facilitate autolytic debridement and rehydration of necrotic tissue.
Iodine	Antimicrobial action
Low-adherent wound contact layer (silicone)	Protection of new tissue growth. Atraumatic to periwound skin Conformable to the body contours
Polyhexamethylene biguanide	Antimicrobial action.
Activated charcoal	Odor absorption.
Protease modulating	Active control or passive control of the wound protease levels.
Silver	Contains silver ions. Antimicrobial properties. Used in infected diabetic foot ulcers or wounds at risk of infection.
Polyurethane film	Control of moisture. Breathable bacterial barrier Transparent therefore allows visualization of wound.
Biological dressings	Collagen or growth factor-based dressings Have components that promote wound healing and tissue regeneration. Used in chronic or non-healing diabetic foot ulcers
Negative Pressure Wound Therapy (NPWT)	Involves application of suction to the wound bed through a sealed dressing system Increased blood flow, reduced edema and enhanced granulation tissue formation. Complex diabetic foot ulcers or wounds with large amounts of exudate.

- *Blood Glucose Monitoring*—Various methods such as fingerstick testing, continuous glucose monitoring (CGM), flash glucose monitoring, HbA1C can be used to monitor blood glucose levels.
- *Medication Management*—This can include oral medications such as metformin, sulfonylureas or insulin therapy. The choice of medication depends on patient's insulin sensitivity, kidney function, and cardiovascular risk.
- *Insulin Therapy*—Different types of insulin (e.g., rapid-acting, short-acting, intermediate-acting, long-acting) can be used either alone or in combination.
- *Dietary Management*—Patients should aim to consume a balanced diet that is rich in whole grains, lean proteins, fruits, vegetables, and healthy fats while restricting intake of refined carbohydrates, sugars, and saturated fats. Carbohydrate counting or glycemic index/load may be helpful for some individuals in managing blood glucose levels.
- *Physical Activity*—Physical activity done regularly helps to improve insulin sensitivity, lower blood glucose levels and maintain a healthy weight.
- *Weight Management*—As excess body weight can contribute to insulin resistance and elevated blood glucose levels, a combination of diet, physical activity and behavioral strategies may be helpful for weight management.
- *Cholesterol Management*—High levels of low-density lipoprotein (LDL) cholesterol, triglycerides, and low levels of high-density lipoprotein (HDL) cholesterol are very common in diabetics which can later on increase the risk of cardiovascular disease.

10.14 Advise to Patient with Diabetic Foot

Managing diabetes is a lifelong journey, and it is normal to encounter challenges along the way. However, here is some advice you might give to a patient struggling with diabetic foot.

1. Wash your feet daily.
2. Dry your feet well, especially between toes.
3. Feel for any bumps or temperature changes.
4. Inspect between toes.
5. Examine each toenail.
6. Check for dry or cracked skin.
7. File toenails straight across.
8. Examine bottom of feet.
9. Track what you find in a record.

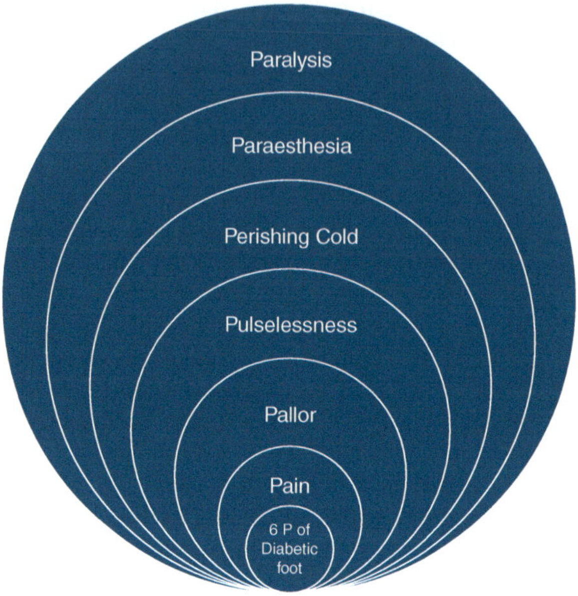

Fig. 10.6 Showing 6 P's of diabetic foot indicating great risk and impending clinical emergency

10.15 6 P's Posessing Great Risk and Impending Clinical Emergency

In diabetic foot ulcers, there are several factors that can pose great risks and indicate an impending clinical emergency (Fig. 10.6).

10.16 Follow-up

Follow-up in diabetic foot patients is crucial for ongoing monitoring, prevention of complications, and ensuring proper management of the condition. The IWGDF 2019 Risk Stratification System and corresponding foot screening frequency [16] helps to categories patients at risk for developing Diabetic foot ulcer. According to these guidelines, the risk category ranges from 0 to 3, representing very low to high risk levels accordingly. Patients are recommended to undergo follow-up appointments ranging from quarterly to yearly, depending on their risk category as above. Major risk factors for these patients include loss of peripheral sensation, peripheral disease of the artery, deformity of foot, history of foot ulcers, lower limb amputation, and end-stage kidney disease.

10.17 Different Stages of Diabetic Foot Ulcer

Any foot deformity in a diabetic patient predisposes them to abnormal pressure distribution, which may lead to vulnerable pressure points prone to injury (Fig 10.7). Over time, a diabetic patient may develop early changes of diabetic foot such as shiny, smooth, wrinkled skin and underlying induration, characteristic of sclerodermoid changes, because of vascular and neurological complications (Fig 10.8). Subsequently, uncontrolled Diabetes may predispose an individual to superficial infection, which may lead to onset of superficial necrosis (Fig 10.9). This progresses to the formation of eschar as seen on the great and second toes (Fig 10.10), followed by superficial gangrenous changes, marked by black, dry, necrotic skin (Fig 10.11). As the gangrene deepens, a trophic ulcer forms at the primary pressure point (Fig 10.12), and autoamputation of gangrenous digits occurs, accompanied by tissue degloving (Fig 10.13). Timely intervention using honey and jaggery dressings initiates a transformation. The treatment facilitates gradual wound healing, showcasing the potential of this approach in managing complex diabetic foot complications (Fig 10.14 and Fig 10.15).

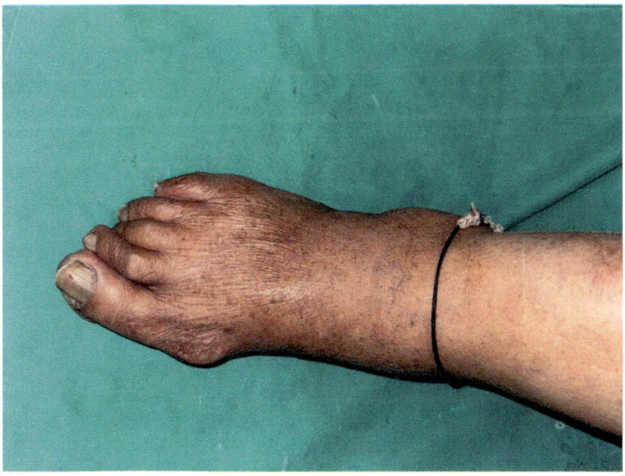

Fig. 10.7 Hallux Valgus joint deformity in a patient with diabetes which later leads to pressure point and ulceration

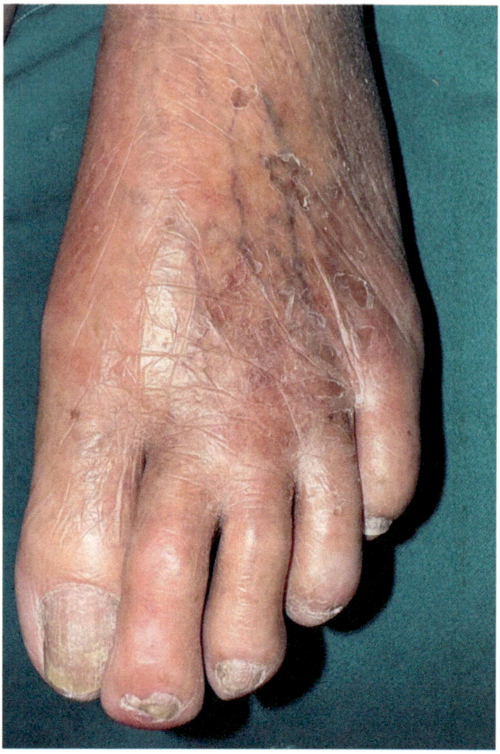

Fig. 10.8 Early changes of diabetic foot (Sclerodermoid changes)—The skin is shiny, smooth, and wrinkled and some induration underlying

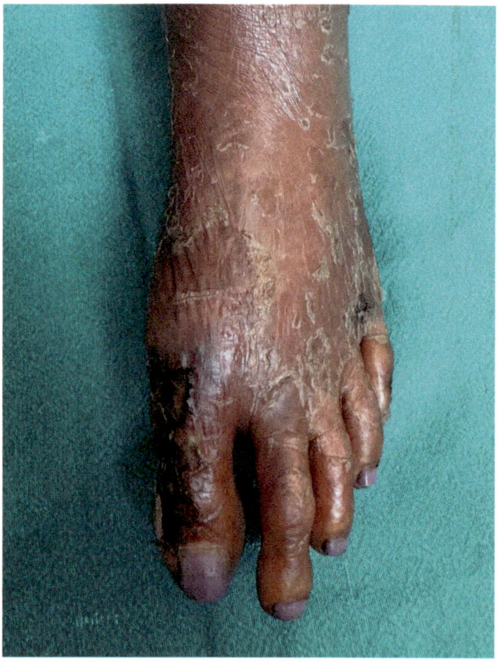

Fig. 10.9 An image of diabetic foot showing superficial necrosis on great toe and underlying fungal infection

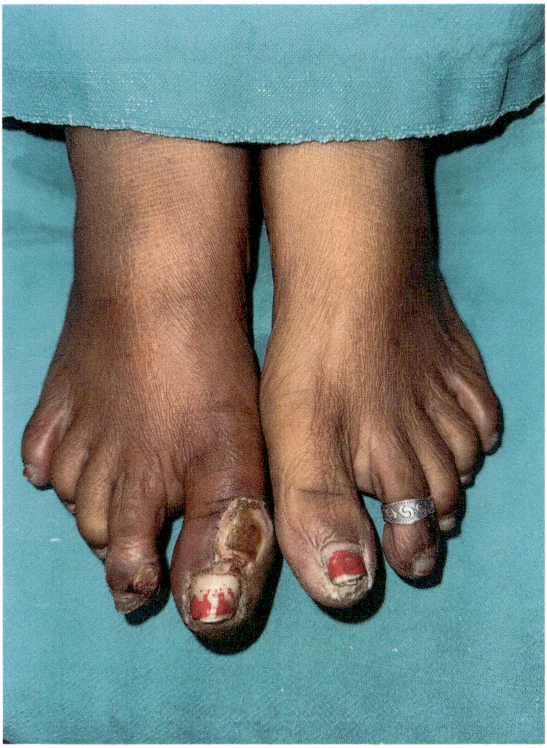

Fig. 10.10 Eschar formation on great toe and second toe after superficial necrosis

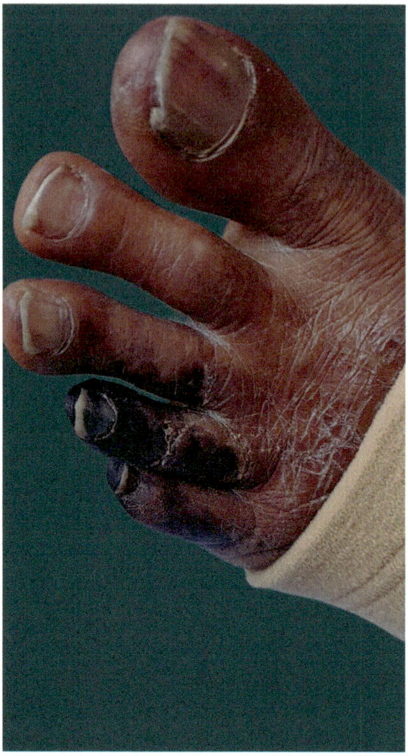

Fig. 10.11 Superficial gangrenous changes showing black, dry, and necrotic skin

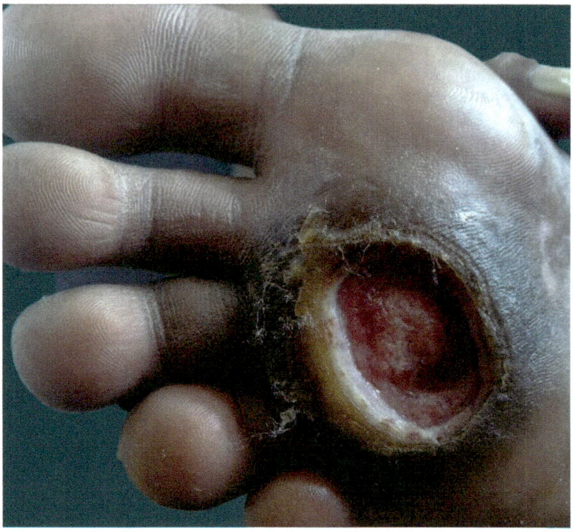

Fig. 10.12 Deep trophic ulceration over the pressure point on foot

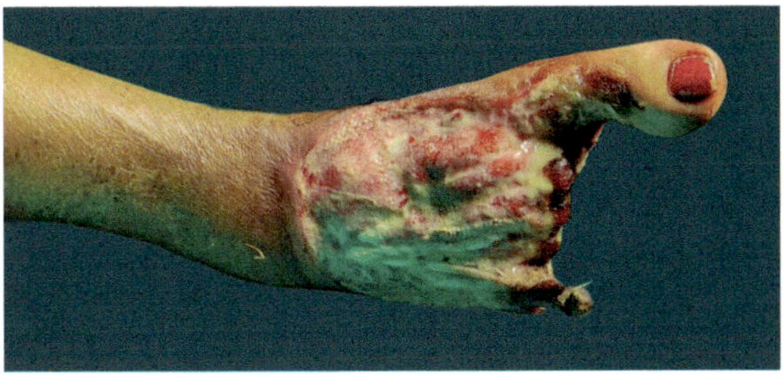

Fig. 10.13 Autoamputation of gangrenous digits with degloving

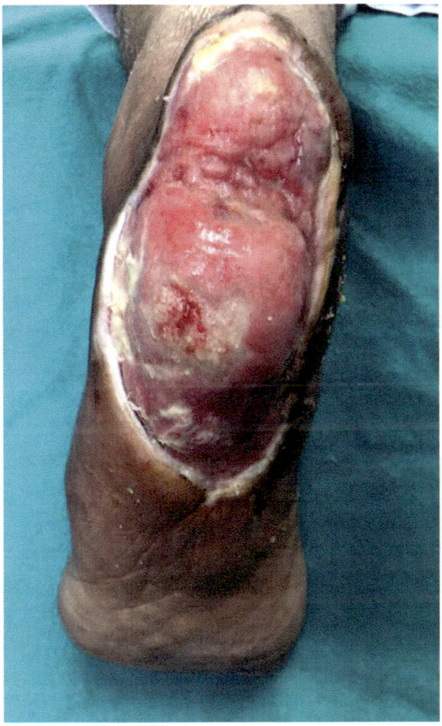

Fig. 10.14 An image of deep ulcer over the calcaneus area of foot before treatment with honey jaggery dressing

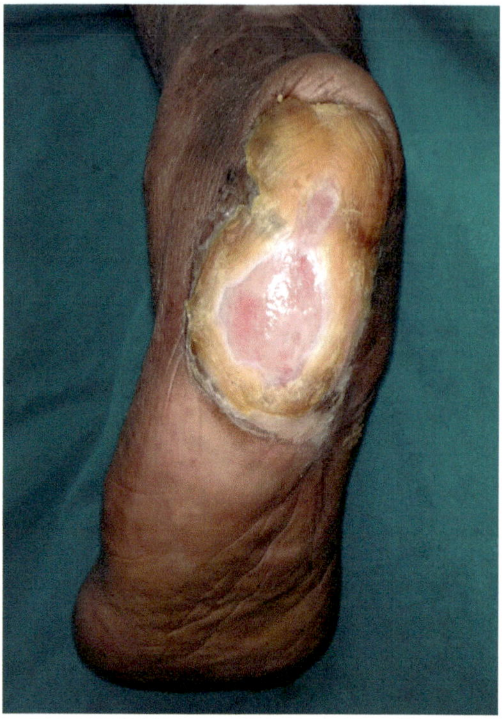

Fig. 10.15 Post-treatment with honey jaggery dressing

References

1. Alexiadou K, Doupis J. Management of diabetic foot ulcers. Diabetes Ther. 2012;3(1):4.
2. Mathers CD, Loncar D. Projections of global mortality and burden of disease from 2002 to 2030. PLoS Med. 2006;3:e442.
3. Armstrong DG, Tan TW, Boulton AJM, Bus SA. Diabetic foot ulcers: a review. JAMA. 2023;330(1):62–75.
4. Neville RF, Kayssi A, Buescher T, Stempel MS. The diabetic foot. Curr Probl Surg. 2016;53(9):408–37.
5. Singh G, Chawla S. Amputation in diabetic patients. Med J Armed Forces India. 2006;62(1):36–9.
6. Raghav A, Khan ZA, Labala RK, Ahmad J, Noor S, Mishra BK. Financial burden of diabetic foot ulcers to world: a progressive topic to discuss always. Ther Adv Endocrinol Metab. 2018;9(1):29–31.
7. Rosyid FN. Etiology, pathophysiology, diagnosis and management of diabetics' foot ulcer. Int J Res Med Sci. 2017;5:4206–13.
8. Kim J. The pathophysiology of diabetic foot: a narrative review. J Yeungnam Med Sci. 2023;40(4):328–34.
9. Armstrong DG, Lavery LA, Sariaya M, Ashry H. Leukocytosis is a poor indicator of acute osteomyelitis of the foot in diabetes mellitus. J Foot Ankle Surg. 1996;35:280–3.
10. Richard JL, Sotto A, Lavigne JP. New insights in diabetic foot infection. World J Diabetes. 2011;2(2):24–32.
11. Wagner FW Jr. The dysvascular foot: a system for diagnosis and treatment. Foot Ankle. 1981;2(2):64–122.

12. Armstrong DG, Lavery LA, Harkless LB. Validation of a diabetic wound classification system. The contribution of depth, infection, and ischemia to risk of amputation. Diabetes Care. 1998;21:855–9.
13. Monteiro-Soares M, Dinis-Ribeiro M. A new diabetic foot risk assessment tool: DIAFORA. Diabetes Metab Res Rev. 2016;32(4):429–35.
14. Acar E, Kacıra BK. Predictors of lower extremity amputation and reamputation associated with the diabetic foot. J Foot Ankle Surg. 2017;56:1218–22.
15. Lipsky BA, Berendt AR, Cornia PB, et al. 2012 Infectious Diseases Society of America Clinical Practice Guideline for the diagnosis and treatment of diabetic foot infections a. Clin Infect Dis. 2012;54(12):132–73.
16. Bus SA, Lavery LA, Monteiro-Soares M, Rasmussen A, Raspovic A, Sacco ICN, Van Netten JJ, on behalf of the International Working Group on the Diabetic Foot (IWGDF). IWGDF guideline on the prevention of foot ulcers in persons with diabetes. Diabetes Metab Res Rev. 2020;36(S1):e3269.

Chapter 11
Diabetic Neuropathy: A Pandora Box in Pulmonary Diseases

Sameer Singhal

Contents

11.1 Introduction

Diabetes is a multisystem disease affecting almost every part of body. Complications of diabetes include macrovascular (coronary artery disease, peripheral artery disease, and stroke) and microvascular involvement (nephropathy, retinopathy, and neuropathy) [1]. As per Kumar et al. [2], diabetes affects 537 million adults globally with 10.5% in the productive age group 20–79 years.

In a recent study done in India by Anjana et al. [3] in 1,13,043 individuals, the overall prevalence of diabetes was 11·4% and prediabetes were 15·3% in the ICMR-INDIAB study between Oct 18, 2008 and Dec 17, 2020. Neuropathy in the distal part, symmetrical in nature is the one of the commonest long-term complications of diabetes affecting more than 90% cases. According to Schreiber et al. [4] polyol accumulation, advanced glycation end products, decreased glutathione levels, and oxidative stress are likely cause of nerve injury in peripheral neuropathy. Tingling, burning, sharp, lancinating sensations typically in night are common symptoms.

S. Singhal (✉)
Department of Respiratory Medicine, Maharishi Markandeshwar Institute of Medical Sciences & Research, Maharishi Markandeshwar (Deemed to be University), Ambala, India

© The Author(s), under exclusive license to Springer Nature Singapore Pte Ltd. 2024

M. Goyal, K. Goyal (eds.), *Rehabilitation in Diabetic Peripheral Neuropathy*,
https://doi.org/10.1007/978-981-97-9290-0_11

11.2 Lungs and Diabetes

Lung diseases are variably affected by diabetes; course of disease, manifestations, outcome are variably affected by presence of diabetes or not. Pulmonary complications in diabetes are referred to as diabetic pneumopathy. Prominent lung conditions affected by diabetes include pneumonia, COPD, overlap syndrome, asthma, tuberculosis, idiopathic lung fibrosis, and lung cancer. Lungs are an important target of diabetes insult as they have a rich blood and nerve supply. It has been observed in various studies that diabetes anticipates the lung aging process and dyspnea and phlegm production are more in type 2 diabetes in comparison to general population of same age, presenting with similar smoking history [5–7].

As per GINA guidelines, a heterogenous chronic disease Bronchial Asthma is characterized by inflammation of airways with previous symptoms like wheeze, chest tightness, dyspnea, and cough with variations in time and intensity, with variable airflow limitation in response to variety of stimuli that provoke little or no airflow limitation in person with no respiratory pathway problem. Dust mites, molds, furry animals, cockroaches, and pollens are common triggering agents. As per Peters et al. [8], one of the asthma phenotypes is associated with obesity with increased IL6 levels and there are high chances of obesity associated insulin resistance. A study by Peters et al. [9] shows that insulin resistance is present in asthma and not related to obesity. Inhaled Glucocorticoids are cornerstone in the treatment of bronchial asthma with less systemic side effects. Oral effects can include dysphonia, oral candidiasis, and laryngeal candidiasis. Systemic administration of steroids causes reduction in the production of ACTH occurs by suppression of hypothalamic pituitary adrenal axis leading to decrease in secretion of cortisols by adrenals may lead to hypoglycemic events.

A study by Kiviranta and Turpeinen [10] concluded that insulin resistance may improve slightly in asymptomatic person after inhalation of high dose glucorticoids, in comparison to decrease insulin resistance and better glucose tolerance in severe asthmatic patients. One should be aware of HPA suppression in higher doses of ICS and increased glucose level due to systemic absorption of steroids and annual screening of HB1Ac and blood sugars can be done in these patients more important in cases who have coexistence of diabetes with asthma.

Watz et al. [11] in a study showed that more than half of chronic bronchitis and COPD patients have coexisting metabolic syndrome with elevation of cells inflammation markers like IL6 and high sensitivity C reactive proteins levels.

ATP 2005 criteria define metabolic syndrome as; presence of waist circumference more than equal to 102 cm (40 inch) in male and greater than 88 cm (35 inch) in females; serum high density lipoprotein cholesterol less than 40 mg/dl in males and 50 mg/dl in females; serum triglycerides greater than equal to 150 mg/dl; fasting plasma glucose more than 100 mg/dl and blood pressure higher than 135/80 mmHg. The main purpose of defining metabolic syndrome is to prevent and keep a watch on development of diabetes in patients of metabolic syndrome [12–14].

According to study done by Falkevall et al. [15], Cui et al. [16] type 2 diabetes is associated with upregulation of molecules that causes chronic structural damage to vascular endothelium such as IL6, angiopoietin (Ang), and vascular endothelial growth factor (VEGF) and downregulation of molecules having protective effect on vascular endothelium.

Lungs have rich microvascular supply. Endothelial dysfunction and increased vascular permeability in diabetes leads to thickening of fused alveolar capillary endothelial cells and basal lamina of alveolar septal epithelial cells. Also, there is reduced amount of tissue plasminogen activator due to increased amount of plasminogen activator inhibitor in intravascular compartment due to diabetes. Tissue plasminogen activator converts plasminogen into plasmin and plasmin in-turn is responsible for fibrinolysis. Therefore, diabetes indirectly leads to increase tendency of thrombosis [17, 18].

Tuberculosis (TB) is a systemic disease affecting almost every organ of body. It can be broadly classified into pulmonary and extrapulmonary tuberculosis. Pulmonary tuberculosis affects lung and is an infectious disease spread by airborne droplet infection, whereas extrapulmonary tuberculosis is generally blood borne, lymphatic or localized extension from primary source and mostly confined to patient [19]. There is three-fold increase risk of tuberculosis with diabetes. TB diabetes patients have more cavitary diseases and are more infective in comparison to non-diabetic tubercular patients due to dysfunctional immunity with hyperactive immune response [20, 21]. There are more chances of reactivation of LTBI (latent TB infection), failure of treatment and reinfection in TB diabetes patients [22]. WHO recommends optimized glucose control as a part of management of TB DM for improved TB outcomes [23].

Idiopathic pulmonary fibrosis is a chronic progressive irreversible lung disease due to unknown cause and is a subset of larger group of diseases called as interstitial lung diseases. It is observed in various studies that prevalence of lung fibrosis and decline in lung function is more in diabetes in comparison to non-diabetic patients [24, 25].

Radiation pneumonitis is most obvious at early stages after treatment and more common in lung cancer patients receiving stereotactic radiation therapy (SBRT) and in patients of lung cancer with diabetes [26]. Type 2 diabetes is a metabolic inflammatory disease with increased level of inflammatory mediators like IL6 and TNF alpha [27]. These inflammatory markers can result in stimulation of collagen synthesis in fibroblast resulting in radiation pneumonitis [28].

11.3 Pulmonary Rehabilitation in Diabetes

Ill-effects of hyperglycemia include dysfunction of microvascular endothelium including arterioles, capillaries, and venules, resulting in decreased nitric oxide availability, increased permeability, and leucocyte adhesion. This further causes insulin resistance and nerve hypoxia especially involving sensory nerves. Long sensory axons in distal limbs are first involved followed by motor neurons.

Physical fitness consists of agility, balance, flexibility, coordination, and power. Aerobic exercises (lowers blood sugar levels, increases insulin sensitivity, reduces triglyceride levels, weight loss), resistance exercises (improve muscle strength), yoga (improves balance and flexibility), weight training (help build lean muscle mass), periodized and non-periodized combined exercises, Tai Chi, inspiratory muscle training, whole body vibration training, and neuromuscular electrical stimulation, all are helpful in restoring physical fitness in diabetes patients.

As per American Diabetes Association (ADA) [29], exercise is a core component of cardiopulmonary rehabilitation program and is a class I indication for management of Type II DM. Increased blood flow during aerobic exercises make more proteins available for ischemic nerve and help in repair of myelin sheath. It also prevents the development of sarcopenia in diabetic patients.

Non-weight bearing exercises should be preferred in diabetic foot. Before doing aerobic exercises, it is important to monitor the blood glucose levels and exercise should be avoided if blood sugar levels are more than 300 mg, as exercise can cause catecholamines with further raise in blood sugar levels, better to eat something before exercises as to prevent catecholamine secretions [29].

Diabetic neuropathy rehabilitation applies to sensorial dysfunction, motor impairment, autonomic neuropathy, and ameliorating pain. Sensorial deficit training start with pressure and pain training followed by tactile and temperature recognition. For motor impairment, rehabilitation program includes passive mobilization of joints for four times a day, later aim is to increase adaptivity for efforts and include walking, climbing upstairs, swimming, etc. Main aim is promoting everyday lifestyle activities which not only have impact on limbs but also improve pulmonary functions as well. Physical exercise reduces autoimmune dysfunction in diabetes and improves various cardiovascular, neurological, sexual, gastric paresis, and sexual dysfunction. Peripheral arterial disease is improved by general measures like stopping smoking, correct glycemia, and antiplatelet treatment. Diaphragmatic breathing, inspiratory and expiratory efforts, deep breaths, shoulder joint movements all are involved in increasing pulmonary capacities in coexisting diabetic patients (Fig. 11.1).

American Diabetic Association [30] recommends both aerobic exercises and resistant training with at least 150 min of moderate to vigorous aerobic activity per week, spread over 3 days per week and two to three sessions of resistance exercises per week on nonconsecutive days.

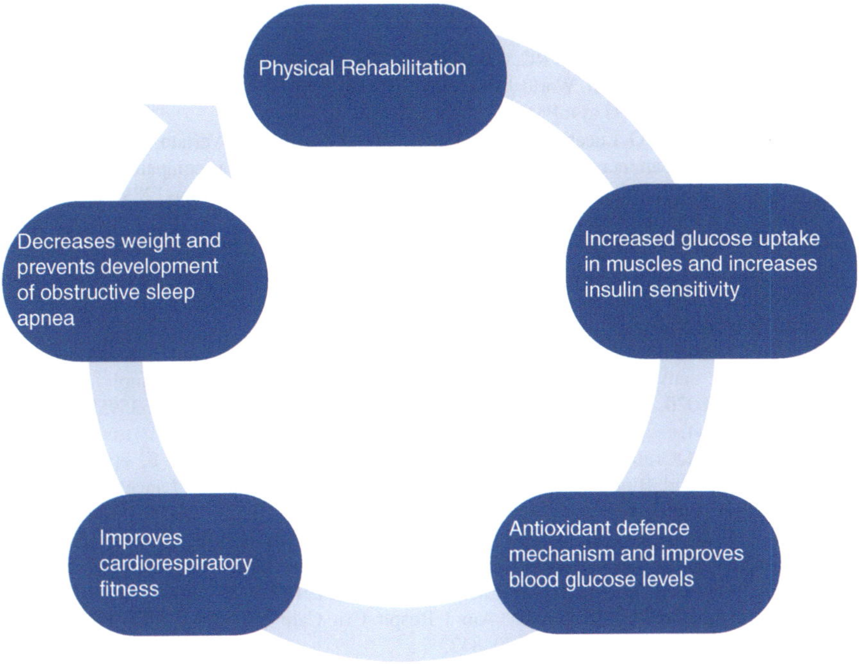

Fig. 11.1 Effect of physical rehabilitation program in patients with diabetes. (Source: self)

11.4 Conclusion

Diabetes and diabetic neuropathy can coexist with various lung diseases and in some of them management of diabetes is essential for the management of lung diseases. Pulmonary rehabilitation and physical exercise in an integral part of treatment of these lung diseases with control of diabetes and prevention of development of diabetic complications including diabetic neuropathies, therefore a pulmonologist should be aware of "diabetic pneumopathy" and how to tackle them with rehabilitation program besides adequate pharmacotherapy.

References

1. Fowler MJ. Microvascular and macrovascular complications of diabetes. Clin Diabetes. 2008;26(2):77–82.
2. Kumar A, Gangwar R, Zargar AA, Kumar R, Sharma A. Prevalence of diabetes in India: a review of IDF Diabetes Atlas 10th edition. Curr Diabetes Rev. 2024;20(1):e130423215752. https://doi.org/10.2174/1573399819666230413094200. PMID: 37069712.
3. Anjana RM, Deepa M, Pradeepa R, Mahanta J, Narain K, Das HK, et al. Prevalence of diabetes and prediabetes in 15 states of India: results from the ICMR-INDIAB population-based cross-sectional study. Lancet Diabetes Endocrinol. 2017;5(8):585–96. https://doi.org/10.1016/

S2213-8587(17)30174-2. Epub 2017 Jun 7. Erratum in: Lancet Diabetes Endocrinol. 2017 Aug;5(8) :e5. PMID: 28601585.
4. Schreiber AK, Nones CF, Reis RC, Chichorro JG, Cunha JM. Diabetic neuropathic pain: physiopathology and treatment. World J Diabetes. 2015;6(3):432–44. https://doi.org/10.4239/wjd.v6.i3.432. PMID: 25897354; PMCID: PMC4398900.
5. De Santi F, Zoppini G, Locatelli F, Finocchio E, Cappa V, Dauriz M, Verlato G. Type 2 diabetes is associated with an increased prevalence of respiratory symptoms as compared to the general population. BMC Pulm Med. 2017;17(1):101. https://doi.org/10.1186/s12890-017-0443-1. PMID: 28716044; PMCID: PMC5513377.
6. Sivgin H, Cetin S, Ulgen A, Li W. Diabetes and bacterial co-infection are two independent risk factors for respiratory syncytial virus disease severity. Front Med (Lausanne). 2023;10:1231641. https://doi.org/10.3389/fmed.2023.1231641. PMID: 38020119; PMCID: PMC10646962.
7. Mizab C, Sánchez E, Gutiérrez-Carrasquilla L, Balsells N, Arqué A, Ruano R, et al. Assessment of dyspneic sensation in patients with type 2 diabetes. Front Endocrinol (Lausanne). 2023;14:1208020. https://doi.org/10.3389/fendo.2023.1208020. PMID: 37635958; PMCID: PMC10457144.
8. Peters MC, McGrath KW, Hawkins GA, Hastie AT, Levy BD, Israel E, et al. National Heart, Lung, and Blood Institute Severe Asthma Research Program. Lancet Respir Med. 2016;4(7):574.
9. Peters MC, Schiebler ML, Cardet JC, Johansson MW, Sorkness R, DeBoer MD, et al. The impact of insulin resistance on loss of lung function and response to treatment in asthma. Am J Respir Crit Care Med. 2022;206(9):1096–106. https://doi.org/10.1164/rccm.202112-2745OC. Erratum in: Am J Respir Crit Care Med. 2023 Mar 1;207(5):636. PMID: 35687105; PMCID: PMC9704842.
10. Kiviranta K, Turpeinen M. Effect of eight months of inhaled beclomethasone dipropionate and budesonide on carbohydrate metabolism in adults with asthma. Thorax. 1993;48(10):974–8. https://doi.org/10.1136/thx.48.10.974. PMID: 8256243; PMCID: PMC464802.
11. Watz H, Waschki B, Kirsten A, Müller KC, Kretschmar G, Meyer T, Holz O, Magnussen H. The metabolic syndrome in patients with chronic bronchitis and COPD: frequency and associated consequences for systemic inflammation and physical inactivity. Chest. 2009;136(4):1039–46. https://doi.org/10.1378/chest.09-0393. Epub 2009 Jun 19. PMID: 19542257.
12. Wilson PW, D'Agostino RB, Parise H, Sullivan L, Meigs JB. Metabolic syndrome as a precursor of cardiovascular disease and type 2 diabetes mellitus. Circulation. 2005;112(20):3066–72. https://doi.org/10.1161/CIRCULATIONAHA.105.539528. Epub 2005 Nov 7. PMID: 16275870.
13. Grundy SM, Hansen B, Smith SC Jr, Cleeman JI, Kahn RA, American Heart Association; National Heart, Lung, and Blood Institute; American Diabetes Association. Clinical management of metabolic syndrome: report of the American Heart Association/National Heart, Lung, and Blood Institute/American Diabetes Association conference on scientific issues related to management. Circulation. 2004;109(4):551–6. https://doi.org/10.1161/01.CIR.0000112379.88385.67. PMID: 14757684.
14. Klein BE, Klein R, Lee KE. Components of the metabolic syndrome and risk of cardiovascular disease and diabetes in Beaver Dam. Diabetes Care. 2002;25(10):1790–4. https://doi.org/10.2337/diacare.25.10.1790. PMID: 12351479.
15. Falkevall A, Mehlem A, Palombo I, Heller Sahlgren B, Ebarasi L, He L, Ytterberg AJ, Olauson H, Axelsson J, Sundelin B, Patrakka J, Scotney P, Nash A, Eriksson U. Reducing VEGF-B signaling ameliorates renal lipotoxicity and protects against diabetic kidney disease. Cell Metab. 2017;25(3):713–26. https://doi.org/10.1016/j.cmet.2017.01.004. Epub 2017 Feb 9. PMID: 28190774.
16. Cui X, Chopp M, Zacharek A, Ye X, Roberts C, Chen J. Angiopoietin/Tie2 pathway mediates type 2 diabetes induced vascular damage after cerebral stroke. Neurobiol Dis.

2011;43(1):285–92. https://doi.org/10.1016/j.nbd.2011.04.005. Epub 2011 Apr 16. PMID: 21515377; PMCID: PMC3096677.0.
17. Chen P. Astaxanthin attenuated thrombotic risk factors in type 2 diabetic patients. J Funct Foods. 2019;53:22–7.
18. Chan K, Chen S, Opdenakker G, El-Asrar AA. Metalloproteinases mediate diabetes-induced retinal neuropathy and vasculopathy. Cell Mol Life Sci. 2019;76:3157–66.
19. Gopalaswamy R, Dusthackeer VNA, Kannayan S, Subbian S. Extrapulmonary tuberculosis—an update on the diagnosis, treatment and drug resistance. J Respiration. 2021;1(2):141–64.
20. Chiang CY, Lee JJ, Chien ST, Enarson DA, Chang YC, Chen YT, Hu TY, Lin CB, Suk CW, Tao JM, Bai KJ. Glycemic control and radiographic manifestations of tuberculosis in diabetic patients. PLoS One. 2014;9(4):e93397. https://doi.org/10.1371/journal.pone.0093397. PMID: 24699457; PMCID: PMC3974751.
21. Behr MA, Warren SA, Salamon H, Hopewell PC, Ponce de Leon A, Daley CL, Small PM. Transmission of Mycobacterium tuberculosis from patients smear-negative for acid-fast bacilli. Lancet. 1999;353(9151):444–9. https://doi.org/10.1016/s0140-6736(98)03406-0. Erratum in: Lancet 1999 May 15;353(9165):1714.. PMID: 9989714.
22. Restrepo BI, Schlesinger LS. Impact of diabetes on the natural history of tuberculosis. Diabetes Res Clin Pract. 2014;106(2):191–9. https://doi.org/10.1016/j.diabres.2014.06.011. Epub 2014 Jul 14. PMID: 25082309; PMCID: PMC4260985.
23. World Health Organization. Collaborative framework for care and control of tuberculosis and diabetes. Geneva: World Health Organization; 2011.
24. Davis WA, Knuiman M, Kendall P, Grange V, Davis TM, Fremantle Diabetes Study. Glycemic exposure is associated with reduced pulmonary function in type 2 diabetes: the Fremantle Diabetes Study. Diabetes Care. 2004;27(3):752–7. https://doi.org/10.2337/diacare.27.3.752. PMID: 14988297.
25. Klein OL, Krishnan JA, Glick S, Smith LJ. Systematic review of the association between lung function and Type 2 diabetes mellitus. Diabet Med. 2010;27(9):977–87. https://doi.org/10.1111/j.1464-5491.2010.03073.x. PMID: 20722670.
26. Kalman NS, Hugo GD, Mahon RN, Deng X, Mukhopadhyay ND, Weiss E. Diabetes mellitus and radiation induced lung injury after thoracic stereotactic body radiotherapy. Radiother Oncol. 2018;129(2):270–6. https://doi.org/10.1016/j.radonc.2018.08.024. Epub 2018 Sep 22. PMID: 30253874.
27. Donath MY, Shoelson SE. Type 2 diabetes as an inflammatory disease. Nat Rev Immunol. 2011;11(2):98–107. https://doi.org/10.1038/nri2925. Epub 2011 Jan 14. PMID: 21233852.
28. Trott KR, Herrmann T, Kasper M. Target cells in radiation pneumopathy. Int J Radiat Oncol Biol Phys. 2004;58(2):463–9. https://doi.org/10.1016/j.ijrobp.2003.09.045. PMID: 14751516.
29. Mensing C, editor. The art and science of diabetes self-management: a desk reference for healthcare professionals. Chicago, IL: American Association of Diabetes Educators; 2006.
30. American Diabetes Association. Standards of medical care in diabetes—2011. Diabetes Care. 2011;34(Suppl 1):S11–61. https://doi.org/10.2337/dc11-S011. PMID: 21193625; PMCID: PMC3006050.

GPSR Compliance

The European Union's (EU) General Product Safety Regulation (GPSR) is a set of rules that requires consumer products to be safe and our obligations to ensure this.

If you have any concerns about our products, you can contact us on ProductSafety@springernature.com

In case Publisher is established outside the EU, the EU authorized representative is:

Springer Nature Customer Service Center GmbH
Europaplatz 3
69115 Heidelberg, Germany

Batch number: 10726135

Printed by Printforce, the Netherlands